Cross
Everything

A personal

journey

into the

evolution

of cancer

Cross
Everything

HENRY SCOWCROFT

For everyone who has ever lost anyone to cancer;
and to everyone who is living with cancer right now.

GREEN TREE
Bloomsbury Publishing Plc
50 Bedford Square, London, WC1B 3DP, UK

BLOOMSBURY, GREEN TREE and the Green Tree logo are trademarks of
Bloomsbury Publishing Plc

First published in Great Britain 2021

A catalogue record for this book is available from the British Library

Library of Congress Cataloguing-in-Publication data has been applied for

ISBN: HB: 978-14729-7512-6; eBook: 978-14729-7513-3;
ePdf: 978-14729-7516-4

2 4 6 8 10 9 7 5 3 1

Typeset in Baskerville by Deanta Global Publishing Services, Chennai, India
Printed and bound in Great Britain by CPI Group (UK) Ltd, Croydon CR0 4YY

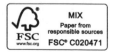

To find out more about our authors and books visit www.bloomsbury.com
and sign up for our newsletters

Contents

Introduction

ALTHOUGH THIS IS A book I never wanted to have to write, I've always loved writing. One of my earliest memories is of posing for a photo for our local newspaper, after winning the £10 prize in a writing competition run by the local library. A decade later, as a biochemistry student, I remember sitting in an intense, cramped tutorial, my tutor's face a picture of bemusement at my latest attempt to crowbar alliteration and assonance into dry academic essays on mitochondrial respiration or bacterial cell division.

But it never occurred to me, back then, that I'd end up as a writer. Instead, I'd chosen to study science thanks to a natural, deep-seated (and occasionally annoying) curiosity about the world around me, inspired by my grandfather, a professor of botany. I'd had aspirations to follow his footsteps into a career in research. But over the course of my degree, as I left behind a string of failed experiments, partially contaminated laboratories and broken glassware, it turned out that writing was by far my strongest suit, and where my future lay. It probably helped that my mother has been, for more years than I can remember, a gardening columnist for a national newspaper, with a quite wonderful turn of phrase. And while she never directly encouraged me into a career in writing, the joy and pride she so obviously takes in wrangling words into her weekly column must have provided some sort of inspiration, even if indirect.

Eventually, it was the urge to marry my two passions – to explain science through the written word – that led me to study for a postgraduate degree in science communication, and which subsequently propelled me into a job as a science writer at a charity: Cancer Research UK, a large, well-loved medical research organisation, headquartered in London. But back then, despite the organisation's long and impressive history – a 100-year-old cancer research charity, the largest in the world – I had no special affinity for or connection with cancer. It was, simply, my first proper job, and one in which I was determined to make a reputation for myself, as someone who could help people engage with and understand the scientific research that had so fascinated me at university.

And so, from the early 2000s until the mid-2010s, I earnestly bashed out a constant stream of articles for the charity's website, on a blogging platform that I and a couple of colleagues set up and managed. As the years went on, they both left the charity to pursue careers as science writers. Both are now published authors in their own right; I always doubted I 'had a book in me', and was content to keep on churning out articles about pretty much every aspect of cancer for the charity's supporters and the wider public, safe in the knowledge that I was probably doing some good in the process.

But that all changed in 2016, when my girlfriend, Zarah, was diagnosed with incurable bladder cancer. Suddenly, out of the blue, my relationship with the disease became personal as well as professional.

One particular memory sticks out, shortly after Zarah's diagnosis. A corridor, and an earnest conversation with a colleague who had survived breast cancer years previously – a gruelling experience, which had had a profound effect on her. 'It's going to be a really rough ride. Find something you love doing, and make time to do it. It'll keep you sane. You obviously love writing – maybe write your way through it?'

I took her advice to heart. I'd already assumed the mantle of keeping our wider network abreast of Zarah's travails via a series of regular emails. As her disease progressed, writing these became a sort of therapy – a way to order the chaos of cancer into something we could cope with, and to use the skills I'd honed over the years writing for Cancer Research UK to reassure, explain, and contextualise Zarah's plight for the many who were deeply concerned about her. Quite frequently – to her occasional frustration – I'd stay up till the small hours, getting the text *just right*, trying to convey our hopefulness and stoicism, explain what might happen next, what the options were. And in the course of those emails, one phrase kept coming up again and again – a plaintive imperative, addressed to the emails' recipients and their inevitable offers of help and support:

'Cross everything.'

As I was to realise, it's a phrase that conveys much about the reality of a cancer diagnosis – something that no amount of blogging about dry academic research papers can teach you. Will the treatment work? What will the scans show? Can we go on holiday? What can I do?

Zarah and I often talked about writing a book about her experience, and 'that's one for The Book' became a bit of an in-joke between us, to be wheeled out in the face of some of the more ludicrous episodes we faced.

We never discussed who'd actually write it. It turned out that it was a job that would fall to me alone.

In the aftermath of her death, several people remarked to me that I 'really should do something' with those emails. The missives had, it transpired, very much hit the mark, revealing to their recipients much about cancer that they'd not known before: the daily grind of the disease's tragic ebb and flow, but also – thanks to the medical and scientific insight I felt necessary to include – something of cancer's underlying nature that many had found helpful. The juxtaposition of the science with the personal seemed vital in conveying both topics.

My decision about whether to adapt these emails, somehow, into a book was further influenced by a small legacy she'd left, in the form of DNA analyses and tissue samples, saved on NHS servers or frozen in anonymous stasis in a freezer in the local hospital. Could these, I wondered, be drawn together to answer questions about her disease: how it originated, what fuelled its growth, and why it was so aggressive. Questions, I suspect, everyone affected by cancer has, but which I was, it seemed, in a position to at least try to answer. And so I set about trying to do so.

Working with researchers to answer these questions has, of course, been a journey of personal closure as much as the substrate for this book; but I hope the answers – and what I learned about cancer along the way – can crystallise, in the book's readers, an understanding of cancer, and that this is, in some way, as helpful for people who read it as writing it has helped me.

So what you're about to read is, in essence, two interwoven stories.

On one hand, it's the story of a tumour, told, as best I can, through careful analysis of Zarah's biological data and that of her cancer. One thing above all else that has fascinated me in all my years writing about cancer is the growing understanding of its evolutionary, Darwinian nature – how, all too often, despite the best efforts of the doctors that treat it, it evolves, adapts, resists and survives. Far from being an inert, uniform ball of cells, researchers are discovering that tumours are dynamic, constantly adapting, ever-changing, battling with the body's defences for supremacy – and are starting to unpick the rules that allow them to do so. I hope the story of Zarah's tumour, and what I've been able to learn about how it evolved, serves as a useful vessel through which to convey this modern view of cancer.

The other story is essentially human: a tale of the life and troubles of a remarkable, compassionate, hilarious, open-hearted woman; one that I hope I've done justice to, and that bears proper testament to the joy she brought so many of us – both before and after her diagnosis – and the impact she's had on the lives of those who knew her.

And although I am in no way religious, I hope that, in some small way, this book passes on something of her remarkable spirit, to live on in – and perhaps inspire – all of you who read her story.

1

Team Twat

I: The mother cell

Scene: The interior lining of a human bladder. A thin, spherical layer of tissue that forms an impenetrable, intricate, elastic barrier – a vital line of the body's defences.

Zoom in: The tissue's surface reveals itself as an endless patchwork of millions of specialised translucent cells, each clamped tightly to its surrounding neighbours, each having graduated from the layers below, and each destined to spend the remainder of its short life locked in a defensive posture, until eventually it withers and dies, to be replaced anew from below.

Pull focus: Stacked beneath the topmost layer lies stratum upon stratum of immature cells, each making a slow journey upwards, to take its place at the surface to mature and fulfil its destiny.

Focus deeper: Sandwiched between the surface layers and a thick external layer of muscle: the vital basal layer. Just a single cell thick, but responsible for everything stacked above it, a continuous font of new life.

Zoom in: Nestled alongside millions of identical neighbours in this delicate layer: a cell. A tiny, unremarkable, disc-shaped bubble of gelatinous life just micrometres in diameter – one among millions. From the outside, all is quiet, the silence belying a hum of invisible activity, the cell's energy devoted, for the last few weeks, to replicating the nearly 2 metres of filament-thin DNA packed into its nucleus with near-perfect fidelity, checking, double-checking, preparing, recharging.

Hold focus. Wait. Watch.

It's here that our story begins.

Suddenly, inside the cell, things spring into life as it starts once more to divide. Each step tightly coordinated and refined by evolution over billions of years, the delicate membrane surrounding its nucleus dissolves while, simultaneously, the nanometre-thin DNA filaments contained within begin slowly to condense into 46 short, stubby chromosomes, each containing two duplicates of a vital chunk of genetic information – thousands of genes held in a few nanometres of chemical architecture. The book of life, in duplex form.

From nowhere, a rigid scaffold precipitates, stretching out across the cell's interior, forming a series of ghostly skeletal tracks that run from one end of the cell to the other.

The disc-shaped cell begins to swell, balloon-like, into a sphere.

Then, like a regiment of soldiers lining up in formation, all 46 condensed DNA chromosome doublets start to assemble across the cell's diameter, perpendicular to the skeleton, each somehow knowing its precise place in proceedings.

Everything in place, the real action begins. Ratchet-like, burning up extraordinary quantities of fuel, the skeleton pushes against itself, forcing the cell apart, tugging one half of each chromosome pair in an opposite direction. The balloon inflates further, and yet more newly formed scaffolding – this time radiating out from the centre to the cell's outer membrane – pulls inward, constricting the membrane around the balloon's centre as if caught in an invisible drawstring.

Slowly at first, then increasingly rapidly, the membrane draws in as the chromosomes segregate – until finally, with all 46 chromosomes safely separated and sequestered into each compartment, the drawstring tightens to pinch the cell clean in two.

The mother cell has a new daughter.

And this newborn offspring now begins the slow migration upwards, away from its mother, towards the surface – programmed to mature into one more building block in the bladder's protective lining.

The mother cell, its job done for now, begins to rest and recharge, readying itself for the next cycle.

But something is amiss. Somehow, at some point during the replication of the cell's metres of delicate DNA, and the wrenching violence of the cellular division, a defect has become embedded in the fabric of its DNA: a submicroscopic lesion that will sow the seeds of a future, unimaginable tragedy.

The exact date of my first encounter with the force of nature that was Zarah Harrison is a matter of some debate, and depends on the exact definition of 'meet'. Both of us belonged to a large, sprawling group of dictionary-definition 'metropolitan elite' types with a healthy appetite for music, festivals, pubs and general late-night hedonism. It was a collision that, given our similarities on so many fronts – not least our love of a cheesy and laboured pun – was bound to happen at some point. It was a surprise to many of our close friends that it took as long as it did.

According to eyewitnesses, the first time we occupied the same room was in the small hours of the Somme-like, rain-ruined Glastonbury 2007, in a mud-infested tea tent. Neither of us can remember this, but apparently it happened.

Then there's the photograph of Zarah on Facebook, at Bestival in 2009 on the Isle of Wight, surrounded, as she so often was, by a multitude of gay men. In a corner of the photo: my cagoule-clad elbow. Zarah had no memory of meeting me there; I vaguely recall bumping into them all while meandering around the festival.

By the time we first recall actually speaking to each other, a year later, in the queue for a boutique music festival, we were certainly aware of one another's existence, if only via the strange and entirely modern phenomenon of being tagged in our friends' social media posts, or otherwise intruding into each other's online lives (I confess, I occasionally clicked through to her profile to find out more about this bleach-blonde so many of my friends knew. Is that online stalking? I suspect it's relatively normal behaviour. But after I confessed this to her, she'd delight in taking the piss out of me as 'a creepy Facebook stalker').

At the time we first spoke, I was with my best friend and housemate, James, who was accompanying me to the festival in part to act as my emotional crutch – I had, just two weeks previously, emerged from a full-on and emotionally draining relationship, and was in a pretty fragile state. I'd almost not gone. As we stood in the queue, James was approached by a striking-looking blonde woman dressed in full pirate regalia, who started chatting to him (he and Zarah had known each other for several years, having travelled together in India and Southeast Asia). Recognising her off Facebook, I elbowed my way into the conversation. Later that day, the festival slowly getting into full swing, a group of us entered a mutual orbit, booze in hand, in the middle of a lawn near the main festival area, and the two of us ended up chatting some more.

Zarah remembered it vividly. 'Every time I looked at you, the background went out of focus. And every time you said anything, I'd laugh. I totally knew then.'

Our orbits collided more fully later that night. Our large group of late-night revellers was infiltrated by a couple of randoms, one of whom had a ghastly Nickelback mullet/ponytail type affair, and who proceeded to make a series of clunky, offensive, mildly homophobic comments. Our group dispersed to get rid of them, agreeing to reconvene at a more secluded area, free of inadvertent bigoted dickheads. Zarah and I, who had by now already progressed from 'highly engaged conversation' to 'occasionally but not so secretly holding hands while no one was looking', headed off into the darkness... only to find Nickelback following us expectantly. We figured the best way to throw him off the scent was to engage each other in a long, passionate snog. It worked.

And so we tumbled joyously into the early stages of what would become the defining relationship of our lives so far. We blagged a lift home from a mutual friend, and made plans to go on a cinema 'date' together the following Sunday. This was unexpectedly brought forward to Saturday night as Zarah, drunk and leaving a friend's wedding, texted me to see if I was still up. I was. She arrived, hammered, at 1 a.m., calling up to me on the balcony, clutching a magnum of champagne, in a bright purple dress with a gregariously frilly red underskirt – a dress that came to define her.

We spent the next day together. I cooked a fry-up for breakfast, and we ate it in bed while reading the *Observer*. A good sign: no competition over the different sections (she went for the Lifestyle and Travel, I for the Comment and Sport – yin and yang already). We eventually made it to the cinema for the late showing. The whole date was us to a tee – late, but we got there in the end.

Over the following months we took things as slowly as we were able, Zarah being unbelievably patient with me as I mended my head after my recently finished relationship. As I healed, our own partnership gradually grew into something profound. In early October we went away together for a weekend in the Cotswolds ('Off cottaging', she'd cackle). On the drive home, I introduced her to an album with which I'd recently become obsessed: Sufjan Stevens' *Come On Feel the Illinoise*. As the chorus to the track 'Chicago' came on, my hand was resting on the gearstick. She put her hand gently on top. That's when I knew.

'Chicago', of course, became 'our' song.

Just seven months later, in May 2011, she moved into my flat in Bethnal Green. It wasn't something we'd planned: her landlord had decided to sell the house she and three of her friends were renting. Although we pretended otherwise, the decision was a no-brainer. James was still living in my spare room; the three of us instantly clicked as a household.

She'd been born in Ireland, in August 1978, in the rainy port city of Cork. The late 70s were not a prosperous time – Ireland's entry into the European Union around six years earlier had opened up the country's traditional manufacturing industry to international competition. Long-established processing factories were struggling, and unemployment was rising. The Celtic Tiger was yet to be born, its roar – which would eventually summon multinational tech and pharma companies to rejuvenate the Cork economy – still a long way off.

Nevertheless, Zarah's parents – Sean, a dashing, charismatic jack-of-all-trades, and Florence, a glamorous former model turned fashion designer – had found a way to provide their daughters – Zarah, and Amber, four years her senior – with an above average upbringing. Around the time Zarah was born, the family moved into a large house in a small residential neighbourhood in the city's north side called St Luke's, where they were to stay for more than two decades.

It was, to begin with, a happy childhood, and Sean and Florence provided a protective environment for the two girls to grow up in. 'We played out in the road,' recalls Amber, 'and always had a nanny, or a housekeeper, to look after us. We were well off by the standards of Cork at the time.' Zarah looked up to her older sister, following her everywhere. 'I sort of hated it at the time, but that's standard big sister stuff, I guess. She always had a kind heart, and quirky habits, paired with a strong sense of independence, and for some weird reason she'd always had this bright red little nose.'

As the girls entered their teens, things between Florence and Sean began to deteriorate. Zarah, something of a daddy's girl, was kept out of the firing line of their blazing rows, unlike Amber, who was 15 at the time. By her account, it was not an easy separation. After a few years of turbulence, Sean eventually moved out, and Florence brought up the girls on her own, taking in students as lodgers to help make ends meet. The family home was sold, and the proceeds invested in a series of properties – Florence switched careers to focus on managing them. When the Tiger finally roared in the early 90s, Florence was in the perfect position to benefit.

Despite religious upbringings themselves, neither Sean nor Florence was especially religious – something of an anomaly in a deeply Catholic country – and this was reflected in Zarah's education, which both her parents took seriously, recognising the value of a good schooling. A spell at a Protestant state school was followed by another at a prestigious Irish-speaking Catholic one. She thrived at neither. But then came one of those moments that becomes the stuff of family legend. Zarah must have told me the story at least 20 times.

Ahead of starting their Leaving Certificates (the Irish equivalent of A-levels), Zarah's best friend at the time, Hannah, was to move to a new school, Newtown – a couple of hours away in County Waterford. Zarah was desperate to join her there, but there was a catch. Newtown was a school founded in the Quaker faith, and only Quaker children could qualify for a free boarding place. But Zarah wasn't deterred – she had a cunning plan. 'My mum was away for the weekend with a friend of hers in Dublin, and Hannah and I hatched a plan to tell Mum that I'd decided to become a Quaker.' On Florence's return, Zarah was desperate to tell her mum the 'news', only for Florence to have some of her own. Reluctantly, Zarah let her mother go first: 'Zarah, at the weekend, my friend took me to one of her Quaker meetings – and it was just so wonderful! So I've got some news. I've decided that I'm going to become a Quaker!'

Zarah and Florence had always had – despite their lack of formal religion – a tendency towards the spiritual and mystical. So when Zarah revealed to her mother her own plans, both excitedly decided that it was no mere coincidence, but something that was somehow Meant To Be. Thus, Zarah's adoption of the Quaker faith was, from the get-go, deep, full and sincere. She started at Newtown a few months later.

By now a charismatic extrovert like her dad, Zarah quickly became popular at her new school, often leading late-night illicit forays into the local town for boys and booze, and generally making mischief. A school friend once told me of her attempted insurrection in the face of an impending vaccination. 'We were all lined up against the wall waiting for our turn, and there comes Zarah, walking up and down the line, fierce as you like, telling all the girls they were *our* bodies and we didn't have to accept it if we didn't want to. None of the teachers knew what to do.'

This rebellious streak and fierce sense of social justice was beginning to manifest itself in other ways. She'd often proudly recall heading up to Dublin, on her own, to join a pro-choice rally – her first such experience. And it was probably in part behind her decision, upon finishing school at the age of 17, to leave Cork to study for a qualification in Fashion Journalism at the London College of Communications.

She arrived in London in 1997 – accompanied by Florence, who'd helped her move over – on the same day that Princess Diana died. Florence recalls pandemonium on public transport, as the UK engaged in a surreal outpouring of grief. Zarah used to joke that the country only had room for one 'queen of people's hearts'.

She took to London instantly. On her first afternoon in halls of residence, Florence fondly recalls her daughter walking up and down the corridor, knocking on doors, assembling a posse for the pub.

Despite always being proudly, patriotically Irish, the city became her home, and she'd often declare that she had no plans to go back to live in Ireland. After getting an NVQ, she started work at a London-based publisher, moved into a flat-share with a bunch of good friends, and set about having as much fun as she possibly could.

II: The mutation

Years have passed. Deep in the lining of the bladder, the damaged mother cell has been robotically, rhythmically, carrying out its duty, division after division, daughter after daughter, its lifetime progeny now numbering millions. Most have since perished, their short lives spent at the front line, clamped tightly together as part of the bladder's protective internal lining, eventually to be replaced from below.

It has not been an easy time. In fact, the mother cell is exhausted. For the last few years, the lining of the bladder – normally home to a symbiotic, peaceful lawn of bacteria – has been regularly invaded by hordes of foreign microbes, outbreeding the natives to establish rampant, unruly colonies. The invaders' presence has called in the cells of the body's immune system – fleets of large, wobbly, bacterium-eating neutrophils, along with specialised secretory cells, whose chemical signals carefully coordinate and control the response to the invaders.

As a result of this ongoing, low-level cellular skirmish, the mother cell has been working overtime to send new daughters to perish on the front line, a routine accelerated by the wash of signals from the immune system. These days, it barely has time to pause and recharge before the next round begins.

And all this time, despite appearing outwardly normal, this particular mother cell, along with all its progeny, have carried a tiny defect in their DNA, introduced during that fateful cell division many years ago. Back then, almost unnoticed, a snippet of information carried on a short stretch of a very long DNA chromosome – the ninth-largest of the 23 pairs in the mother cell's nucleus – was accidentally deleted. Lost along with it were instructions to assemble a particular protein molecule, a small part of a complex machine honed by millions of years of evolution to govern whether the cell that contains it should divide – a go/no-go system designed to keep everything in regular order.

Each time the mother cell produces a new offspring, this tiny defect – in a tiny part of its multilayered control system – is passed on. Consequently, though imperceptibly, a small patch of the bladder's defensive lining is now made up of ever so slightly abnormal cells, all descended from their ever so slightly mutant mother.

Yet, so far, this solitary genetic deletion has had minimal consequence: those same evolutionary millennia have conspired to ensure that, in the nucleus of every cell in the bladder – including the mother cell's – resides a second copy of this lost information: each of the cells' chromosomes has a life partner, a subtly different sibling with which it has cohabited in the nucleus ever since the mother cell's distant ancestor was first formed in a womb long ago, after egg and sperm first fused.

And so, despite the loss of this tiny info-snippet – a genetic recipe for a small but vital cog in a larger control system – the back-up copy allows the mother cell, and its daughters, to function safely and normally.

Until today.

Once more, just as it has countless hundreds of thousands of times before, the mother cell gears up for another exhausting round of division, activating microscopic molecular machines to crawl along all 2 metres of its 23 chromosome pairs, sucking in simple molecular building blocks and fusing them together, to painstakingly create an exact copy of each in its wake.

Normally, as with every one of the mother cells in the bladder, a multitude of error-correction mechanisms ensure that this division is a near-flawless process, introducing at most a handful of minor, inconsequential errors across the billion letters of molecular code contained in the cell's DNA genome.

But today, just as the cell's replication micromachinery arrives at the remaining, working copy of the control gene… once again, by awful, tragic coincidence, something inexplicably jams, twisting and breaking the DNA strands, shearing the precious molecule in two.

Immediately the machine seizes up. Molecular alarms ring out. The entire process of DNA replication in the mother cell grinds to a halt, and more cellular control systems kick in to try to rectify the situation.

Sensing the error, the cell activates yet another molecular machine to rescue the situation – a DNA editing machine. This tiny DNA editor locates the chromosome's twin, spools to the region bearing the long-since deleted control switch – and uses it as a template to try to patch up the fractured DNA.

The cell, of course, has no consciousness, no motive, no awareness of what it is doing, of the irreversible error it's making.

Mechanically, faithfully, it transcribes the region bearing the missing information over to the second chromosome. In doing so, it hard-codes the control gene's loss forever into the cell's genome. A vital cog in the cell's control system has just been irretrievably deleted – overwritten in error. The mother cell now is a second step along its catastrophic journey. A cellular car with its brakes gently, imperceptibly damaged – if not, yet, snipped entirely.

But for now, the immediate crisis is over. The replication of the mother cell's imperfect DNA is complete. And just as before, all 23 duplicated chromosome pairs – two of which are now imperceptibly shorter – condense and line up. The cell's internal skeleton assembles, the cell balloons, the invisible drawstring tugs its membrane inwards – and everything is wrenched apart once more.

By mid-2011, Zarah and I were fully coupled-up, comfortably cohabiting and getting to know each other's extended networks. For Zarah, this included a tight-knit group of female friends accrued during her years in publishing – and a constellation of gay men who, since everyone else was busy breeding, very quickly became a big part of our social lives (I'd go weeks without seeing a straight man outside of work). For me, this included a wide network of friends I'd collected while playing music in bands throughout my 20s, some very close friends from work (Zarah became a regular at our post-work pub sessions) and a tight-knit group of friends from my university days. Previous girlfriends had occasionally struggled with this latter group – Zarah, however, fitted in as if she'd been there from Freshers' week.

We were in our mid-30s, happy and settled – even if we did quickly acquire a reputation for being both horrifically late for everything and also the last to leave. These were characteristics we'd both had individually; combined, we enhanced each other's disorganised superpowers tenfold. We summed up our shared bacchanalian fecklessness with a self-deprecating nickname – 'Team Twat' – that later on we'd whisper to each other, with an accompanying hand-squeeze, when things got tricky.

Team Twat decided very early on not to have kids – a decision that always raised an eyebrow among our be-kiddled friends ('Oh, is there something, you know... wrong?', one cheerfully asked, upon learning of our barren intentions). It was an easy choice to make – both of us had our own reasons but we shared the main ones: namely an anxiety over passing on the baggage from our difficult childhoods, and a love of a good hungover lie-in. As well as sidestepping these crucial issues, it was a relief not to have to worry about the practicalities of incomes, house sizes, school catchment areas, etc. Life was simple, fun, and happy.

As well as getting to know each other's broader groups of friends, we also met each other's families, always a milestone in any new, serious relationship. My first trip to Cork was particularly memorable. We'd intended to fly late on a Friday after work; however, events conspired to have us miss our flight ('events' as in we were engrossed in a crossword in a bar in Stansted airport – *so* 'Team Twat'), so we had to check into a hotel near the airport and get up at 4 a.m. to ensure seats on the first Cork-bound Ryanair flight. So when we arrived, we were shattered. Zarah's mum, Florence – a wonderful, chaotic whirlwind of a woman, who adored and doted on her daughter – met us at the airport and announced that the homeless charity she helped run was to be filmed for TV that day, and would we mind helping out as, effectively, extras – starting in a few hours. So my first experience of Cork family life was to chop a mountain of carrots while trying not to fall asleep on camera, surrounded by charity volunteers and homeless people. The rest of the day was somewhat less stressful, and culminated in a lock-in in the local pub with Zarah's dad, Sean, playing cards and drinking Beamish until about 2 a.m. But the real pièce de résistance happened the following day, as Florence insisted that we accompany her to her local Quaker meeting.

In the car on the way to the meeting house, I sat silently in the back seat nursing an enormous hangover, as Zarah and Florence chatted in the front. It emerged that, as well as the usual hour's silent reflection, Florence had somehow become involved in putting on some sort of memorial tree planting after the service. The trouble was, she couldn't remember who it was for. 'How about Mrs Y?' Zarah asked. No, Florence said, she's still going strong. Well, how about Mr X? No, he died ages ago. This game of 'Guess the Dead Quaker' continued for some minutes, to be brought to an abrupt halt by Florence's mobile ringing – it was another of the Quakers, Natasha, asking Florence if she'd like to lead the tributes. Bluffing, still driving, she quickly declined and said it would be far better if someone else were to do it. The call ended, and nothing further was said about the matter.

In the wood-panelled meeting house, in a brief spell of glorious sunshine, I had my first experience of Quakerism: an hour's silent reflection. The 60 minutes came and went, and I absolutely loved it. An hour, no phones, no newspapers, no radio, in tranquil silence – my mind wandered around all sorts, and I saw why Zarah would often remark that it was her special time to solve the little things in her mind that had been bothering her. I was pretty taken with the whole thing, and by the time the hour was up, I felt almost transcendentally relaxed. So I was far less alert to what followed than Zarah.

As agreed in the car, Natasha stood up and announced the tree-planting memorial, and that she'd be saying a few words about how the awful loss must have affected Florence's family, how it was so wonderful that Florence's daughter Zarah and her partner, Henry, were here so soon after Zarah's miscarriage, and how the unborn child would live on through the tree to be planted in its memory.

All eyes swivelled to us. Zarah froze, open-mouthed. As the penny dropped, Florence looked slightly embarrassed. 'No, no, it was my other daughter, Amber! She had the miscarriage! Sorry, everyone!' I was still too blissed-out to cringe, but the look Zarah gave her mother was something to behold.

After a quick, barely calming cup of tea, with Zarah still fuming ('Mother!' she'd hissed under her breath. 'Amber's not even a Quaker!' 'She came to a meeting once!' 'What, that time she sat outside in the car? That doesn't count!'), the congregation all trudged out through the resuming standard-issue Cork drizzle to the cemetery behind the meeting house. There, in front of a tall drystone wall, a hole had been dug, next to which stood a potted fig tree, adjacent to a plaid-shirted gardener who had just finished digging it. We stood in silence as he sombrely removed the tree from its pot and placed it in the hole. Then, first Florence was summoned forward to shovel in a spade of earth, followed by a scowling, furious Zarah. Finally, it was my turn. Barely 48 hours after meeting Zarah's mother and father for the first time, I was paying Quakerly tribute to her sister Amber's unborn child. I hadn't even met Amber yet.

To cap things off, the gardener passed round some dried figs to eat while we had a further few minutes' silence. The collective squelching and chewing perfectly captured the absurdity of the proceedings. At the end of the silence, perhaps out of awkwardness, Florence addressed the crowd: 'Thank you very much, everyone!' she said, waving like Queen Elizabeth

'Get in the car,' hissed Zarah.

So yes. That was my introduction to the batshit insanity of Zarah's wonderful family.

Meeting my mum proved to be a much less dramatic affair than my trip to Cork – and she and Zarah got on from the instant they met. We even introduced my mum to her mum; they formed an instant bond based, in part, on poking fun at the pair of us – they were like a female version of Statler and Waldorf, the two old men in the balcony in *The Muppet Show*. This led to several joint family Christmases, one in Ireland (Zarah, Mum and I hired a cottage near Amber and her husband, Michael) and two in the UK, both on the South Coast. It was something both of us had always craved – stable, relatively drama-free family time, with both of us there for each other to deal with the inevitable stresses as they arrived. And although we never made it out to stay with them in Brussels, my dad and his wife, Joelle, also met Zarah several times on their trips to the UK.

I cannot stress how much this mutual familial acceptance and love meant to both of us, particularly after our parallel fragmented, high-stress childhoods. And, of course, it was support that became utterly vital after Zarah got ill.

Music played a big part in our relationship – none more so than the music of Sufjan Stevens, the American singer-songwriter whose music I'd been infatuated with long before meeting Zarah, and with whom she also fell in love. On my 34th birthday, in May 2011, Zarah took me to see him play the second of two shows at London's Royal Festival Hall. I was over the moon – even more so when we subsequently discovered that one of her friends, Kesh, had two spare box tickets for the first night too. Being mildly obsessed with him by now, we went to both. But oh my word, that first night, magically suspended in a box to the left of the stage, his neon-encrusted multi-musician extravaganza blew us away, reducing all four of us – me, Zarah, Kesh and her friend – to tears by the end of the set, 'our' song, 'Chicago', culminating in a huge balloon drop on to the audience below us. And as he delicately sang the refrain – 'All things go' – we held hands as happy tears ran down our cheeks.

On the bus home that night, Zarah snoozing on my shoulder (she could sleep *anywhere*), my phone buzzed as an email newsletter from Stevens' record label arrived in my inbox, announcing an end-of-tour show in Prospect Park, Brooklyn, NY – tickets for which were a mere $15. The date, early August, was near enough to Zarah's birthday for me to immediately, reciprocally, book two (to hell with the cost of the air fare). I kept it a secret, for a bit.

August eventually came, and we spent a long lazy week tramping about Manhattan before it was Sufjan-time again. He didn't disappoint – and once again closed the set with 'Chicago'. This time, instead of balloons, huge, transparent beach balls were ejected into the audience from backstage, to be bounced in the air over and over by the crowd. Zarah, of course, wanted one as a souvenir. Obviously, getting it past security would mean deflating it. So, after the set finished and everyone melted away into the night, Prospect Park was treated to the silhouette of Zarah straddling a giant beach ball, squeezing it with her legs, while I held the valve open and tried to coax the air out of it. More than once we had to dash off as the security guards prowled with their torches.

I still have that beach ball. It now resides in my spare room, in a large paper gift bag stuffed in a corner, along with a whole collection of other ephemera and artefacts Zarah collected as mementos of our travels and adventures. I haven't looked in it since she died. I still can't.

Over those five years we were together, our relationship grew and blossomed. Despite our large and dispersed friendship group, and our almost hyperactive social lives, we had become best friends as well as lovers. We did pretty much everything together. I remember the shock when, after nearly a year living together, Zarah headed to Australia for a few weeks to be joint best man at her friends' wedding (always one with the gender equality, was our Z). It was the first time we'd spent more than a few nights apart since she'd moved in.

And despite the fact that I'd worked for a charity for years, she also introduced me to my first proper taste of front-line charity volunteering, as she convinced me to sign up as a driver on the Quaker Mobile Library for the homeless, which she'd been volunteering on for years. Despite my grumbles about the oft-early weekend starts, we had a huge amount of fun, and got to know several of the other volunteers and borrowers extremely well – so well that, after she died, several of them came to pay tribute to her at her memorial.

III: The guardian

The damaged mother cell struggles on dutifully, churning out daughter after daughter, supplying its local patch of the bladder lining as best it can.

But its behaviour is subtly different. The loss of the 'go/no-go' control switch genes has made it impatient, failing to pause and recharge sufficiently between divisions, instead hurriedly attempting to divide before its chromosomes are fully duplicated and aligned on the cell's skeleton.

It has also developed a stutter. Every so often, as the cell uncoils and then replicates its chromosomes, the micromachinery occasionally repeats short sections of genetic information – a molecular stammer with the potential to amplify the information hard-coded into each subsequent daughter.

To begin with, most mistakes are inconsequential – duplications of short stretches of DNA that contain little that is relevant, at least for the mother cell's primary job: spawning new cells to maintain the bladder's protective lining.

But things are going downhill. The cell has become reliant on sophisticated fail-safe mechanisms, molecular control systems programmed to patch together incomplete chromosomes, unravel tangled DNA strands, and otherwise ensure everything is as close to normal as possible before the next wrenching division.

At the heart of these overarching control systems is an ancient evolutionary relic: a molecular guardian that first arose nearly a billion years ago, now present inside every complex cell on Earth. Should the impatient mother cell make too great an error, its own internal guardian stands poised to trip the alarm of all alarms: a cellular suicide switch baked into the very genetic design of life itself. The guardian is, to borrow a phrase, a backstop to a backstop.

And yet – like every component of the cell's multiple fail-safe mechanisms – the guardian, too, is vulnerable: tucked away on a short stretch of DNA on one of the cell's smallest chromosome pairs, the instructions to make it are encoded in the very DNA it exists to protect.

Years ago, the loss of that tiny control switch was the first step on our cell's fateful journey. Now, today, the events that unfurl are, decisively, the second.

First, during another hurried round of division, as the mother cell's replication machinery reaches the segment of the chromosome that bears the guardian's DNA code, it makes another unforced error: a single rogue, uncorrected typo, a fateful mistake in the order of building blocks that encodes this fundamental information.

From now on, whenever the mother cell uses this garbled template to replenish its supply of guardian proteins, they're misshapen, broken and hyperactive – both unable to function as nature intended and, by a freak of biology, now possessed of strange, unnatural powers, allowing them to activate long-dormant programs encoded in the mother cell's DNA. Its behaviour becomes yet more erratic, as does that of all its progeny.

And as the errors continue to build up in the cell's DNA, with almost inevitable tragedy, another mistake occurs during another round of cell division. While duplicating the guardian's remaining 'normal' back-up copy, the cell stumbles once more. The gene is irreversibly corrupted, and the cell is forced to overwrite it – using the mutant version on the other chromosome.

With these two simple mistakes, the guardian itself has become irreversibly corrupted. The fail-safe has failed. From now on, each of the mother's daughters bear this deranged, faulty cellular software, and each is now free to grow and divide unchecked. Nature's brake cable has now been decisively cut. The distinction between mother and daughter has entirely broken down. If one were to look from one to the other and back, it would be impossible to say which was which – a lineage of defective cells driven to proliferate out of turn, uncontrolled.

And so each impatient, stammering cell exponentially becomes two, becomes four, becomes eight, becomes sixteen… and gradually, from this small patch of the bladder's lining emerges an ever-expanding clump of millions of proliferating, impatient, unruly cells – mere millimetres in diameter but massive in consequence.

Of course, it wasn't all sunshine and stars – although I had a stable, satisfying job, Zarah was all at sea, career-wise, and this put a fair bit of strain on our relationship. The roots of this began a year or so before we'd met, when Zarah jacked in her blossoming career in publishing to go travelling in Asia and South America, returning to unemployment and the dole. Zarah used to joke, with characteristic inappropriateness, that I was dating the *Daily Mail*'s worst nightmare: an immigrant benefit-scrounger from a nation of terrorists.

Over the subsequent years, Zarah struggled to get a full-time job, bouncing from temp post to temp post, sometimes on the reception desk of large fashion houses, sometimes at digital publishing start-ups, before winding up in 2012 as a marketing executive at Tesco's clothing label, F&F. Their offices were located a horrible hour-plus two-train commute away in bland, soulless Welwyn Garden City, for which Zarah had to get up at 6 a.m. Further salt was rubbed in the wounds by having to leave me dozing peacefully and smugly in bed for a couple more hours before I made the 20-minute bus ride to work up the road in Angel. This contrasting routine, quite understandably, infuriated her – both because she was consistently knackered (once so much so that she fell asleep at the table while we were out for dinner with my dad), and also because I had a tendency to work late and get home full of beans just as she was winding down for the evening. She also, frankly, hated the job, hated being on a temp contract, hated not doing something she was passionate about, and hated working for a company that was, at the time, in the news for all the wrong reasons – including selling people horse-meat under the guise of mince (I bought her a T-shirt off the Internet with the Tesco logo spelling out the word 'Horse'. She never wore it. Good boyfriend skills, Henry).

She toyed briefly with the idea of training to be a counsellor, working with homeless or drug-addicted adults, and volunteered briefly for a couple of organisations. But despite her work with the Quaker Mobile Library, the fact that she 'only' had a vocational NVQ, rather than a bachelor's degree, ruled her out of all master's courses; scraping the funds together for a three-year undergraduate course seemed like an unattainably long slog. I thought at the time that this was nothing short of a tragedy – she would have made an incredible counsellor. You could see it in the way she interacted with people while doing library shifts – she was non-judgemental, open, warm, friendly, and a fantastic listener, and possessed of the most acute emotional intelligence of anyone I've ever met. At a time where such skills are so needed by so many, the barriers thrown up in her way were almost criminal.

Thus, although everything else in our lives was pretty much idyllic, the mismatch between our working lives (and thus our ability to seriously plan for the future) was causing tensions, and there was no resolution on the horizon. So, to fix things, we did what any grown-up would do... and ran away.

In truth, we'd been talking about going travelling ever since we first got together – but Zarah's discontent at Tesco (and the fact that she'd managed to scrape together some meagre savings) really brought things to a head. I asked for, and got, a six-month sabbatical from Cancer Research UK (I'd been there for exactly a decade, so my request was quickly accepted), we booked some tickets, sublet my flat to a close friend, and headed off into the unknown.

It was all the clichés – a holiday of a lifetime, mind-expanding, etc., etc. We literally circumnavigated the globe. We started in St Petersburg, got the train all the way through Russia and Mongolia to Beijing, then flew to Southeast Asia, where we spent three months visiting Malaysia, Thailand, Burma and Singapore, before flying to Australia for Christmas and the Boxing Day Test Match (dream come true), then finally heading to South America for another three months, via Chile, Argentina, Bolivia, Colombia, Ecuador and Brazil.

Throughout my life, I've always found it a truth that travel makes or breaks relationships – usually the latter. It made us. During those months, and its attendant scrapes and adventures, we grew even closer – something neither of us imagined possible. Zarah was, unsurprisingly, an amazing, unflappable travel companion; I didn't do so badly either, although I did have the occasional flap when plans changed at short notice (irritatingly, Zarah would accuse me of 'channelling my mother'). We arrived back in the UK, relaxed, smug, tanned, happy, in March 2014, and picked up precisely where we left off, but even more tightly bound.

———

I slotted back easily into the team at Cancer Research UK, where it felt like nothing much had changed (they certainly hadn't found a cure). Zarah began the search for a job, secure in the knowledge that, despite having blown all her savings (and a chunk of mine), she had a roof over her head, a stable, loving partner, and all the time in the world to find a job she loved – the one missing piece in an otherwise perfect partnership.

Frustratingly, it took several false starts and unhappy rejections, and almost a year, for that 'something' to arrive, during which time the post-travelling glow had worn off and Zarah's mood and confidence slowly degraded once more. It came thanks to a chance comment at lunch with a long-term friend and former colleague of Z's, Erin, who was now a senior executive at Marks & Spencer (it was actually Erin's wedding that Zarah left to come to mine for our first 'date' four years previously). Erin's team was looking for a digital marketing manager for the company's food products – a new role for a slightly old-fashioned but well-regarded organisation struggling to adapt to the new online world – and, having seen her in action in previous jobs, she was convinced Zarah was a good fit for the role.

However, Zarah – confidence rock-bottom – took some convincing. 'She's only doing it because she feels sorry for me!' she told me, in an uncharacteristic bout of self-pity. 'That's complete bollocks,' I remember saying. Erin – a strong, brilliant, hyper-intelligent high-flyer who had previously won awards running the *News of the World*'s marketing team – was emphatically NOT the sort of person who'd put her reputation on the line, suffer fools, or open herself up to accusations of cronyism. Go for it, I told her. Go. For. It.

She went for it, nailed it, and never looked back.

It was a whole new Zarah. At M&S she got to travel, to plan, to strategise, to unleash her creativity – a side of her that, save for brief bursts for friends' birthdays or Christmas decorating, had lain hidden from me for as long as I'd known her. She wowed the exec board. She smashed her targets. She took on more and more responsibility. The talk was of hiring new people for her to manage, of expanding the team. It was joyous to watch – and it's heartbreaking to know that none of that will ever happen. Because just as she was happy, content, and confident. Just as we let our guard down and dared to think about moving house, getting a dog, doing all the things we only dared dream of. Just after a wonderful Christmas with our mums and our best friend, Lindsey. Just as we hit peak happiness. Just then. The bomb went off.

Just then, she found out she had advanced, incurable cancer, and everything changed forever.

Life really is a fucker, isn't it?

Here comes cancer

IV: The doubling

Scene: The lining of a human bladder.

Zoom in: A small clump of spherical, disordered cells, no more than a few millimetres across.

Hold focus. Things are about to take a turn for the worse.

As each of these odd, spherical cells gears up for a new round of division, yet more catastrophic genetic events occur as they try to replicate their jumbled, muddled chromosomes in slapdash, make-do fashion.

Frequently, these catastrophes are just too much for the resulting progeny to bear – their DNA is too far from normal, too fractured, for their remaining alarm systems to ignore. Despite the missing guardian, the cells self-destruct, shedding debris far and wide. Sensing something amiss, nearby immune cells – already present in the bladder lining in large numbers, recruited by the now frequent bacterial rampages – mobilise to try to contain the damage, migrating to the site of the anomaly and amassing at its edges.

Gently, carefully, the immune cells extend their tiny molecular sensors, stroking the forest of molecules on the surface of each rogue cell, looking for outward signs of aberration. Alas, despite their odd behaviour, their scrambled DNA and their impatient, rapid growth, as far as the immune system is concerned, each of the rogue cells still 'feels' just like every other cell in the bladder.

Nothing to see here. Move along.

And so, ignored by the immune system, the mass continues to grow unhindered.

Time passes. And just occasionally, the random nature of events conspires to confer new, ever more lethal superpowers on the cells of this growing, expanding mass.

Zoom in: Deep within the growing mass, one cell has, as is usual, duplicated its 46 now mangled chromosomes in preparation for another division. Ninety-six chromosome pairs line up on the central scaffolding, poised and ready. But as the cell gears up to divide... something snaps. Rather than separating equally – 46 for each offspring – all 96 are pulled to one end of the cell. The drawstring pulls tight. A monster is born.

This monster bears twice the normal machinery, twice the potential for rapid growth, and twice the buffer against catastrophic loss of another essential component.

It gradually outgrows its siblings, the resulting horde forming the bulk of the growing mass.

Then, later, within this rapidly expanding mass, more chaotic, stuttering cell division ensues. Inside one of the monsters, as it gears up to divide anew, uncoiling and copying its metres of error-strewn DNA, the internal copying machinery again stammers: a large stretch of DNA is inadvertently replicated first once, then twice, then again... until four copies are present, end to end – a molecular stammer with profound consequences. Quite by chance, this repeated stretch of DNA contains instructions to make microscopic molecular antennae, honed by nature to sit in the cell's external membrane. In normal times, their job is to sense delicate hormone-like signals in the cell's environment and, upon doing so, execute a host of internal programs in tightly regulated fashion.

But these are not normal times.

With the antenna gene quadruplicated, the monstrous cell coats itself with hundreds of thousands of molecular aerials, becoming hypersensitive to the background noise of growth signal. In turn, these grossly amplified signals now instruct the cell to activate long-suppressed software, profoundly influencing not just its own behaviour, but those of its surroundings, in myriad ways.

If the effect of earlier calamities – the lost control switch, the scrambling of the guardian gene – was to cut nature's brakes, now this hyperactive signalling presses a foot on one of its accelerator pedals. The cells' rapid growth and unruly behaviour accelerates anew, shifting into an even higher gear.

> Thus, unnoticed – step by random, chaotic step – in this small region of the bladder's lining, a tiny clump of cells has finally – lethally – become transformed.

It was a cold, dark, rainy January night in London. I'd just left work to play my regular Wednesday night squash game with my friend Bob – and I was running late. Standing in the drizzle at a bike rental post, repeatedly, frustratedly jabbing the buttons on its insensitive touchscreen, trying to actually rent one of the bloody things, my phone rang. 'Not now, Zarah,' I thought, as I answered, still jabbing at the touchscreen. But then I heard the panic in her voice, and stopped. 'Hi, it's me, Zarah.' She always, always, started calls like that – even to me, even with her name on the screen – but today she sounded different. 'I've had some bad news. It's my dad. He's not well.' Back in Cork, Sean had been rushed to hospital with acute pneumonia, and was in intensive care.

Of course, Sean – a lifelong 20-a-day smoker and perpetual fixture in his local boozer, Carroll's – had had run-ins with ill health before. His circulation was slowly packing up, his fingers were stained brown, and he had a wheezing smoker's cough. So we'd expected something bad to happen one day. But what was freaking Zarah out was the memory of a particularly hairy encounter a decade or so earlier, long before we met. Then, a mysterious, acute brain condition saw Sean's entire system rapidly deteriorate, to the point that, when Zarah's aunts collected her at Cork airport, she was told it was too late. She wept in the car all the way to the hospital.

Yet by the time they arrived, things had taken a Lazarus-like turn for the better. Sean's systems were rebooting; he was regaining consciousness. It was a miracle; the doctors were baffled. He went on to make a full physical recovery (although, Zarah said, he was never quite the same again). The cause was never identified, but the usual suspects – aneurysm, stroke, infection – were all ruled out.

For Zarah, as a perpetually late person, the painful memory of believing she'd missed her dad's departure had haunted her ever since.

So this time she was determined to get over there as quickly as possible. The trouble was, the first practical option was an early flight the next morning – the day's last departure was in 45 minutes, there was no way she'd make it, and an agonising, fretful evening lay ahead.

In the rain at the bike rental station, I realised I should probably cancel squash. 'Do you want me to come home now?' 'Yes please,' she whispered.

At home, I helped Zarah pack. The complicating factor, although we didn't yet know quite how complicating, was that she wasn't in great shape herself either: she was taking antibiotics for yet another painful urinary tract infection. They were the bane of her life – she'd suffered from them since she was in her late teens. Apparently, it was 'something to do with the shape of her bladder'. In 2010, she'd had a cystoscopy (a camera inserted down your wee-hole... You may now uncross), which, apparently, showed no signs of serious abnormality. She'd been allowed to keep the photos, which she proudly showed me soon after we got together. 'Aren't they pretty? It looks like a star system or something! I've got a galaxy in my bladder!'

This time, as with a previous flare-up last October, the infection had spread to her kidneys, and she was in considerable pain. The antibiotics hadn't yet kicked in, so she needed constant paracetamol. I was worried about her flying.

'I'll manage.'

She always managed. She *hated* making a fuss about being ill.

To take her mind off things, we cuddled on the sofa as we caught up on Season 5 of *Game of Thrones*. At the time, rumours were swirling of its creator George RR Martin's ill health. 'I hope he doesn't die before he finishes the bloody thing,' Zarah quipped once – a comment that resurfaced in my head, unbidden, years later, as I started watching Season 7. It's not as much fun, watching it on your own.

She left for the airport at dawn the next morning. We'd agreed that I'd stay behind for now – things were pretty full on at work as the team prepped for a big, complex science story we were putting out – a breakthrough in understanding how the immune system could, potentially, be trained to target cancer. I was leading on producing a whizzy CGI animation explaining it all (we'll come back to the significance, and coincidence, of this later). But I'd promised to be on the first plane out, should things deteriorate further.

Over the weekend Sean's condition stabilised and, happily, he started to pull through. Zarah decided to stay on until he was safely back home. Meanwhile, her kidney pain had been getting worse, not better.

The following Wednesday, she texted me at work – a simple 'Can you call me please?' Something wasn't right. I called. That morning, she'd gone to the loo and a huge blood clot had come out in her urine. 'Seriously, it was enormous. It made such a splash! Freaked me right out – I thought a rat had jumped in the bowl or something!' We agreed she'd go to her mum's GP the next day – Florence booked her an appointment.

But that afternoon, while visiting her dad in intensive care, still really worried and in pain, Zarah took herself down to the Accident & Emergency unit. After a few hours' wait, she was eventually seen... only to be sent away with yet more antibiotics.

I can't remember who decided that, despite the verdict from A&E, the trip to the GP was still a good idea – but Zarah kept the appointment. The GP, sensing something was seriously wrong, sent Zarah back to A&E, but to a different hospital – one with a fully fledged urology unit. A CT scan was ordered, and she was kept in overnight while the specialists examined the results.

As she told me shortly afterwards: 'I remember thinking to myself, I'll know if it's something serious if the next thing I see is a consultant marching down the corridor towards me, white coat billowing out, flanked by a couple of juniors – like on *ER* or something.'

That's exactly what she saw next. The scan had revealed a *something* – a mass – in her bladder, blocking the entry from her right ureter (the tubes that pipe fresh urine down to the bladder from the kidneys). Her kidney was blocked and swollen and full of wee – hence the pain. The blockage could be one of a number of things – it could be a kidney stone. It could be inflammation from the infection. It could be...

...well, it could, but that would be hugely unlikely in someone so young.

She called me at work to deliver the news. Afterwards, I hung up, calmly crossed the office, crouched down next to my manager's desk, shaking, and asked if I could take the next day off – Zarah had an 'abnormality' in her bladder. I needed to fly to Ireland.

I booked a flight, for 7 o'clock the next morning, and a room in a hotel next to the hospital. Florence collected me from the airport. The next few hours are a blur. Florence's terrible parking. Zarah's cheery demeanour hiding her panic inside. The walk up to urology for another cystoscopy. Waiting alone in the corridor outside. The map in the corridor, of local confirmed urological cancer cases in County Cork (just… why??). The tears running down her face as I walked back in the room.

'They think it might be cancer, Henry.'

Fuck. Not her. Not us. Fuck.

Sharing a cup of tea and two stale biscuits on the ward as we waited to see the specialist. The fireplace. Why would a ward room have a fireplace? The specialist – lovely, but clearly worried too, explaining the immediate course of events: the probe with the camera used for the cystoscopy wasn't designed to do much more than take pictures. Zarah would need to have a process called a 'TURBT' (a 'trans-urethral resection of bladder tumour') to take tissue for analysis. This was basically an operation under general anaesthetic, with a much more robust probe, able to remove the mass. Would we like it here? Or back in London? They could schedule it in for a couple of weeks.

The decision was simple to make: we'd fly back to London and look to have the procedure there. But thank you. Zarah was discharged, and the three of us – Zarah, Florence and I – had lunch in a café over the road from the hospital and tried, calmly, to parse these events, and plan a way forward. We were all being very stoic, the mood deflated but not sad. I cancelled the hotel room – we would stay with Florence that night, and fly back to London the following morning. While we ate, Zarah booked flights; I sent an email from my phone, to Cancer Research UK's then chief clinician, Professor Peter Johnson – a marvellous, kind man with a wonderful dry wit and a calm, reassuring wisdom, known affectionately as PJ, with whom I'd worked closely over the years – saying, basically: 'Help.'

Then I excused myself, went to a toilet cubicle, and punched seven kinds of shit out of the wall.

———

Back at Florence's that evening, mid-dinner, my phone buzzed: Peter had emailed back, offering sympathy, help, the recommendation of Professor John Kelly at University College London Hospital (UCLH), and the advice that Zarah should visit her GP in London ASAP, and get a letter of referral. Seconds later, he emailed Prof Kelly and copied me in.

Despite the gathering storm clouds, both Florence and Zarah were hugely relieved – even excited – to know things were in hand, with the top experts on the case. That night, in Florence's spare room, in darkness, with Zarah curled up exhausted next to me, even though I knew I shouldn't, I looked up on my phone everything I could find about bladder cancer.

It's fair to say I didn't really like what I found out.

We flew back the following morning. It was a bright sunny day. I can remember looking out the window at the vivid green rolling Irish countryside below us as we took off. We held hands for the whole flight.

Prof Kelly emailed back the next day. 'Of course, I'd be happy to help.'

Zarah saw her GP on Monday morning, got the referral letter, then got straight on the Tube to UCLH to hand directly to the team there, along with a CD-ROM of her scans from Cork.

They booked her in for the procedure for the following week.

It had begun.

I think it's probably worth spending some time dwelling here on exactly what I – at that exact moment – understood by the word 'cancer'. After all, I'd been writing about it for more than a decade – my accumulated knowledge was the prism through which I – and by extension, Zarah – viewed everything that happened next.

Of course, every popular work about cancer – whether it's a memoir, a science book, a feature article or whatever – must, inevitably, at some point, drop into an expository section about what the disease actually is – usually beginning with the clichéd words 'cancer starts when the cells of your body divide out of control'. I've written this phrase countless times over the years – indeed, my very first task all those years ago, as a young communications graduate learning the ropes at Cancer Research UK's London HQ, was to write a whole new section for the charity's website called, appropriately enough, 'What is cancer?' So it's a section of this book I'm approaching with trepidation – it's such well-trodden terrain that I fear this may be unutterably dull, or repetitive, or clichéd. But it needs doing, for two reasons. The first is obvious: to try to really get to the heart of Zarah's story – to understand what had happened in her bladder and everything that followed. But I also want to bring you up to speed with what, by late January 2016, after a four-year biochemistry degree, then 14 years writing about cancer, of conferences, interviews, reading papers and the like, I understood about the disease with which Zarah had just been diagnosed.

So let's start with a paradox: like so much in medicine, a great deal of what we know about how our bodies work, whether it be mental, physiological, molecular or cellular, is derived from the study of what happens when it goes wrong – in other words, from studying diseases like cancer. But on the other hand, the best way to *explain* what cancer is – its true, brutal nature – is to first start by describing how 'normal' life works. Some of this might be old hat for those of you who've studied biology beyond your mid-teens – feel free to skip ahead if so. For the rest, let's start at the beginning, and think about the idea of *control* – particularly, control of what happens in your body, and when.

You began when a single fertilised egg in your mother's womb started to divide. One cell became two; two became four; four became eight, and so on. That single microscopic speck became an embryo became a foetus became a baby became a child. Became you.

But today, as you read this, you're far more than a ball of identical cells – you've grown into a vast array of different specialised tissues and organs, all of which originated from that initial dividing clump, but which now is able to, for example, sense the light bouncing off this page and interpret these words into meaning. It's pretty incredible, when you think about it – your ability to read this book is because, decades ago, several of those cells 'decided' to make your eyes. But after that initial growth spurt, what's truly remarkable about our bodies is how, once the basic plan has been established – eyes, limbs, teeth, brains and the rest – this hive of activity slows right down: once your eyes become eyes, they (usually) stay eye-shaped and eye-sized. Whatever instructions your cells used to make you you, they obviously have a built-in 'stop' mechanism – they somehow 'knew' when they were in the right place, with the right neighbours, doing the right jobs.

Of course, we're not completely fixed in time and space – over the days, months and years, things get worn out and damaged. So almost all of our tissues have the ability to self-renew. This is especially true of the bits of us that are exposed to the rest of the world – our skin, the lining of our lungs, mouth, stomach, bowels and bladder and our reproductive systems. But as well as these obvious sites of renewal, the replenishing of our cells happens all over the place. Our liver cells get worn out as they remove toxins from our blood. And our bone marrow constantly produces new blood cells to replace those that get knackered as they race around through our arteries hundreds of times an hour.

But, Goldilocks-like, all of these tissues have to regenerate at exactly the right pace – too little would be bad; too much and, well… that's cancer. But let's not leap too far ahead – let's stick with 'normal' for now. What I'm trying to get across here is the idea of an extremely sophisticated, extraordinarily tightly regulated control system, operating both within our cells and throughout our tissues, keeping us just the right amount of alive.

A particularly beautiful example of this is the way you heal after a cut.

When your skin is broken, the damaged and dying cells release signals to their neighbours, triggering a highly ordered cascade of events. First, nearby blood vessels constrict, slowing any bleeding; meanwhile, tiny blood-borne cell-like blobs called platelets are triggered to stick together, starting the formation of a blood clot.

Minutes later, with a clot in place, the bleeding staunched, new signals are sent out, causing the surrounding tissue to become inflamed – the blood vessels open up again, allowing nutrients and oxygen to flood the area, and a whole family of different types of immune cell arrive on the scene, to clear up the debris and engulf or destroy any invading bacteria.

Then the real magic begins. Blood clotted, debris cleared, the skin cells at the edge of the wound – which, for the majority of their lives, have just sat there, protecting you, maybe sweating a bit, maybe making some hair – kick into action and start multiplying and moving. Over the next couple of days, they grow in number to cover over the wound, forming a scar. Cells called fibroblasts pump a protein called collagen into the region, binding the new skin cells together to form new tissue. Blood vessels branch out and grow into and through the damaged region, supplying the new cells with blood and oxygen. Eventually, the new tissue – now made of skin cells, fibroblasts, blood vessels, pigment cells and a host of others – forms an almost perfect bridge across the wound. Then, finally, once everything is in place, the signals switch yet again, and the process winds down. The inflammation abates. The wound is healed. Of this extraordinary cascade of processes, only a small scar remains.

It's taken researchers decades to unpick the basics of this healing process, to understand the nature of these 'signals' (in reality, complex protein molecules secreted by a variety of different cells in the skin and blood), their timing, where they come from – and, despite everything that's been discovered, it's still not fully understood. Anyway, I hope this little anecdote serves to illustrate the idea of control, on a cellular level, and how phenomenally intricate it is. Any misstep on this pathway – the inability to clot, the failure to kick-start new blood vessel growth, a blunder in flipping the final 'off switch' – and you could be in serious trouble.

Which brings us to cancer.

Most people, I suspect, know that 'cancer = too much growth', and have a vague idea that a tumour is made of 'cancer cells' that are growing too fast, and spreading. But this idea, of the 'cancer cell' as the rogue entity causing the disease, much like the HIV virus causes AIDS, or *Salmonella* bacteria cause food poisoning, is vastly, incredibly oversimplified. Although rogue, multiplying cells are, as we shall see, a hallmark of the disease, there's much more to it than that. A tumour is the consequence of *a loss of control* in a region of tissue in one of the organs in the body. As we'll see, a growing tumour needs more than rapidly multiplying cancer cells – it needs a new blood supply; it needs to co-opt the immune system to nurture it rather than attack it; it needs fuel to generate energy. In short, far more than a clump of rogue, aberrant cells, a tumour is a small, rogue *organ*, growing and dividing in the body, subverting the usual control mechanisms one by one – *evolving* – and causing havoc as it does so.

So, how do cancers arise? How do the shackles of control, normally so tight, get broken with such devastating consequence? To understand this, we once again need to revert back to talking about 'normal' biology. We need to zoom in a level and take a look at what genes and DNA are, how they work, and how they control and coordinate the behaviour of the cells and tissues of your body.

Pretty much every one of the 200-odd different types of cell in your body – from the neurons in your brain to the germinal cells that make your toenails – contains a central structure, visible down a microscope, called a nucleus. And it's here that the cell's DNA molecules – known as chromosomes – are found.

DNA – which is an abbreviation of its chemical name, DeoxyriboNucleic Acid – is a long molecular chain of many millions of smaller molecules called nucleotides (or sometimes, 'bases'). There are four types, called adenine, thymine, cytosine and guanine, which, for simplicity's sake, are usually referred to by their first letters: A, T, G and C. This means all sorts of literary metaphors abound when discussing genes and genetics. Changes in a cell's DNA become 'typos'; we talk of genes being 'transcribed' and 'translated'; we even refer to DNA being 'the book of life', or its 'instruction manual'. But even though metaphors can be helpful, sometimes they can be a distraction – DNA is not a book, and nucleotides aren't letters.

DNA is, in fact, an extremely stable molecule, and this is why nature selected it to hold the master copy of the instructions a cell needs to run. These instructions are 'written' (sorry) in the order of nucleotides that make up the DNA and – here's the nifty fundamental bit – this order specifies the order in which to assemble another, rather different, set of building blocks: those that make up a different type of molecule – proteins.

It's hard to overstate the importance – and beauty – of this simple, elegant fact of life: that one molecule – DNA – contains the instructions for building another – proteins. And so before we press on with DNA and genes, here are a few things to note about proteins.

The components of a cell that actually 'do' things, and make up the bulk of life as we know it, are (almost) always proteins. The keratin that makes up your hair and nails, the haemoglobin that carries oxygen round your blood, the albumin in the white of the egg in the omelette you had for dinner in front of the TV, the amylase in your saliva that broke down the carbohydrates in the bread you ate with it while you watched *Big Brother*, the collagen that that awful chap had pumped into his lips these are all different types of protein, each with a specific job to do. And just as DNA is made of chains of nucleotides, so proteins are chains of molecules called amino acids. There are 20 or so amino acids that occur in nature, and it's their precise order in a protein that determines its biological properties.

So, back to DNA. As we've seen, the order of amino acids in a protein (or to use the more scientific word, its 'sequence') is determined by the sequence of nucleotides in a given stretch of DNA. Hence, you'll often hear of DNA being 'sequenced' – this is just a fancy term for analysing (or even 'reading') the exact order of nucleotides it's made of, and thus, what protein it makes. Not all DNA sequences are capable of making protein, and it turns out that hardly any of the 2 metres of DNA in each of your cells contains protein-building instructions (although it seems to do a number of other things, as we'll see in a bit). So, given the importance of these protein-coding regions of our DNA, we have a special word for them.

We call them 'genes'.

For example, the DNA in human cells contains two sequences that specify the order in which a cell must join together amino acids to make one of two separate proteins, known as α-globulin and β-globulin. Once made, these two proteins pair up to form the oxygen-carrying protein we call haemoglobin. And so we often, simplistically, say that a gene 'makes' a protein (although the 'making' is a somewhat more complex process, as we'll see below). Even more simplistically, sometimes we say that a gene is 'for' a particular trait, such as red hair, or cancer. But it's worth remembering that a gene is only ever 'for' a protein. The trait itself is the consequence of what that protein does.

Right, we're getting there, but there's an anomaly. DNA is made of long strings of just four nucleotides, but proteins are chains of amino acids – of which there are 20 types. How does nature use a four-letter code to carry information about the order of amino acids in a protein? How do four 'letters' in one language get translated into 20 in another?

It turns out, as a cell 'reads' the information encoded in DNA, it does so three letters at a time. In other words, each amino acid is 'spelt out' by a sequence of three DNA nucleotides. This is the famous 'genetic code', and deciphering it is one of humanity's greatest achievements. In almost every organism on Earth, for example, a sequence of three cytosines in a row – CCC – is the code for one particular amino acid (one called proline), while the triplet 'AAG' tells a cell to include another, called lysine.

I'm not going to dwell too long on this triplet code, how it arose over millennia, and why it's so cool (although believe me, it's absolutely fascinating), save to make this point: if a single nucleotide in a gene's DNA sequence is somehow replaced by another (a single-letter change, to stick with the typographical metaphor), it can change the amino acid it specifies – and this, in turn, can cause the resulting protein to do something unintended. Which can have profound consequences.

To illustrate this, let's consider an example beloved of biology textbooks – an inherited blood disorder known as sickle cell anaemia, which is, in essence, a disease of the β-globin gene. In people with this disorder, a particular three-letter sequence right near the start of this gene has a single 'letter' difference – a thymine rather than an adenine – so it reads GTG, rather than the normal GAG found in most of the rest of the population. This causes their blood cells – as they make haemoglobin – to put an amino acid called valine in place of the 'correct' one, called glutamic acid. The resulting protein has a disturbing property – when the blood's oxygen levels get low, it clumps together into long strands inside red blood cells, killing them. Thus, when someone with sickle cell anaemia exercises, and their blood oxygen levels plummet, their red blood cells have a nasty tendency to self-destruct. One single nucleotide difference, resulting in a dramatically different experience of life.

OK, that's DNA, genes, proteins, and the genetic code. A few more key concepts to cover, then we will, I promise, get back to the matter in hand.

First: chromosomes – the giant DNA molecules magically packed into each cell's microscopic nucleus. Chromosomes are no ordinary DNA molecules – they've been carefully honed by evolution both to carry information and be replicated faithfully whenever a cell divides. Perhaps surprisingly, as I mentioned above, most of a chromosome *doesn't* contain genes – instead, they're dotted along its length, interspersed with vast stretches of DNA whose function researchers are still understanding. Some of this code plays other roles – regulatory switches, a central structure called a centromere that's essential for cell division and, at each end, structures called telomeres that act like the little plastic caps at the end of your shoelaces, preventing the whole thing from fraying. But a lot of it is still quite mysterious in function.

The exact number of chromosomes in a given cell differs from species to species, but whatever the number, the entire complement of chromosomes is known as an organism's 'genome'. The human genome is made of 46 chromosomes, thus every human cell (except sperm and eggs) contains 46 of them. Dogs' cells contain 78. Earthworms' genomes have 36. Whatever the species, it's always an even number, and this is basically because of sex: half of your chromosomes come from your mother, the other half come from your father. So, more accurately, a human cell contains 23 *pairs* of chromosomes – and thus, two copies of every gene (forming a handy back-up mechanism should something go wrong).

A particular gene's location on a given chromosome is essentially constant in a given organism's genome – for example, in every human being, chromosome 11 (i.e. the 11th longest human chromosome) contains, at a precise location on one end, the β-globin gene mentioned above. (This turns out to be pretty handy, as it means researchers can use the same genetic 'map' for every human being.)

Chromosomes are, in molecular terms, absolutely massive: they're typically made of about 100 million DNA letters, and the total human genome contains about 3 billion – an almost unimaginable number. So as well as posing a fearsome challenge to scientists as they tried to work out how to sequence it, this vast length also poses a formidable challenge to a cell itself: as I've mentioned before, the nucleus of a single human cell a few micrometres in diameter contains about 2 *metres* of DNA. That's quite a packing problem.

Thankfully, it's a packing problem nature has solved elegantly. In a living cell, the long, thin chromosomes are wound round millions of tiny packing proteins called histones – nature's own bobbins – to form a dense, highly ordered DNA-protein gloop called chromatin. In a given cell, only a tiny fraction of its genes will be needed at any one time – active DNA is in an unwound state, but the rest is tightly stashed so as to avoid damage.

Right, we're into the home stretch of this bit of biological mansplaining, so now on to the final important set of concepts: how does DNA actually *work*? How is it replicated and repaired, how do genes 'make' proteins, how are they switched on and off, and how does this affect how a cell behaves?

To get your head around this, I need to briefly touch on a fundamental property of DNA that I deliberately skipped earlier. Each of the four nucleotides – A, T, G and C – has a particular affinity for just *one* of the others: adenine loves sticking to thymine, while cytosine pairs with guanine. As a result, chromosomes are, in fact, made up of two complementary DNA strands. One bears the genetic information, while its partner forms a protective mirror image – and these twist around each other like a rubber ladder, each 'rung' a pair of nucleotides, to form the famous double helix discovered by Francis Crick, James Watson, Rosalind Franklin and Maurice Wilkins in 1953. It was a discovery that paved the way to what we now know about how genes work (as we'll see next), and also – crucially – how DNA itself is replicated: this ability to pair with one – and only one – other type of nucleotide means each strand carries the instructions to make its mirror image. When DNA is copied, tiny molecular protein machines work their way along each strand, gradually building up a new, complementary strand using the existing one as a template.

This exquisite ability to encode and direct its own replication is also the secret underlying a cell's ability to repair damage to its DNA – something that happens on a near-daily basis. Minor damage to one DNA strand can be patched up using the information on the other. And larger-scale damage, affecting both strands, can be repaired by using the information on the chromosome's twin – the second copy, inherited from your other parent.

Our genomes contain a multitude of different replication and repair systems – many of which go rogue in cancer and are, as you can imagine, the source of intense focus for cancer researchers.

But replicating its information is merely one challenge facing a cell. Another is how to read it and make use of it.

The process of 'reading' a gene to make a protein begins in the nucleus, when a section of DNA is unwound from its histones, the two strands separated, and their nucleotides exposed to tiny, sophisticated protein-based transcription machines (themselves, of course, products of genes). These machines bind to a specific 'start' sequence at the beginning of the gene, and move along the DNA strand. As they do so, they use the sequence of nucleotides to construct a complementary strand of a subtly different chemical called RNA – a molecule very similar to DNA, but much less stable.

Upon reaching the end of the gene, the transcription machinery releases this newly formed RNA copy of the gene, and the process begins again. Meanwhile, each newly created RNA molecule finds its way out of the nucleus and into the cell's main compartment – the cytoplasm. Here, fiendishly complex molecular translation machines called ribosomes grab the beginning of each RNA molecule and, finally, use it as a template to build the protein encoded by its nucleotide sequence.

So, in a short space of time, a single active gene can be used to make millions of RNA copies of itself, each of which can be read multiple times by the tens of millions of ribosomes in the cytoplasm. In this way, a cell can rapidly make vast quantities of a particular protein, should circumstance so dictate.

But what are these circumstances, and how can they 'dictate'? To explain this essential concept, we're going to have to simplify things, with a worked example that's relevant to cancer (see, we're getting there). Let's zoom out of the nucleus, through the cytoplasm, and look at the outer surface of the cell.

A typical cell is covered in a whole range of molecular sensors – each a protein encoded by genes – which allow it to respond to its environment. One such sensor is made by a gene that encodes instructions for a protein called the 'epidermal growth factor receptor' (abbreviated to *EGFR*). After being made by the cell's ribosomes, the EGFR protein* makes its way to the cell surface, where it floats around, embedded in the membrane, with a sizeable portion protruding out into the cell's exterior, and a smaller portion sticking into the cell's interior.

As its name suggests, EGFR has evolved to sense the presence of a hormone-like protein called epidermal growth factor (which, as you might have guessed, is abbreviated to EGF), which certain tissues can secrete under particular circumstances. When EGF reaches a cell bearing the EGFR sensor on its surface, it sticks to it, causing the portion of EGFR protein inside the cell to undergo a chemical change that – in a process not dissimilar to that desk toy with the dangly balls, Newton's cradle – sets off a chain reaction inside the cell.

First, the activated EGFR molecule causes particular proteins in the cytoplasm to also become activated. In turn, these activate a cascade of other proteins, which activate yet more proteins called transcription

---

*A short note about gene and protein names: The accepted convention, which I have used for this book, is to italicise gene names, but not the proteins they produce. Hence, '*EGFR*' refers to the gene that makes the protein EGFR.

factors, which ultimately find their way into the nucleus. Some of them bind to particular stretches of chromosomes, causing them to be unwound at that specific location and the genes they contain to be transcribed. Others do the opposite, deactivating previously active genes.

The genes ultimately affected by signals from EGFR include those that regulate cell division – so when EGF binds to it, the net effect is that the cell starts to grow and divide (hence EGF being described as a 'growth factor').

This is, of course, vastly oversimplified, but I hope you get the basic principle – that particular environmental cues can, by affecting the activity of different sensor proteins, trigger a cascade that switches multiple genes on or off, changing the suite of proteins a cell is making, and thus altering its behaviour.

I chose *EGFR* as an example, but there are thousands of different sensor proteins encoded by our DNA (not all of which are on the cell surface – many, for example the receptor for the hormone oestrogen, are found in the cytoplasm). And not all the cues and stimuli are external – for instance, our cells can respond to high or low levels of internal building blocks or nutrients, or changes in pH, and adapt accordingly. Similarly, our vast chromosomes also encode thousands of signalling molecules – the middle balls in the Newton's cradle – that pass on signals like those from EGFR, and thousands of gene-activating transcription factors. And – because nature *really* loves to give biochemists a challenge – it turns out that these signalling pathways have a considerable degree of crosstalk. Even just beginning to work all this internal wiring out has taken decades, and whenever I think too hard about how complex it all is, I feel simultaneously awestruck and headachy.

Right. That's the basics of life distilled into a few thousand words.

Let's talk about what happens when the whole thing fucks up.

Let's talk about cancer.

In January 2000, two American cancer researchers, Doug Hanahan and Bob Weinberg, published an essay in the scientific journal *Cell* that would go on to become one of the most referenced works on cancer in human history. In it, the pair summarised nearly 100 years of cancer research, trying to answer the question of what, exactly, are the disease's defining features. They called these the Hallmarks of Cancer – which was the essay's title. (I have an obscure, tangential and slightly nerdy personal connection to it: nearly a decade ago, in 2011, while on a Wikipedia training course, I wrote the Wiki page summarising their article, which itself has gone on to be widely linked to, translated and cited.)

I'd first come across the 'Hallmarks of Cancer' essay a few months before that, while listening to Doug Hanahan give a keynote address at a research conference, to mark the article's 10th anniversary year. By that time, I'd been at Cancer Research UK for about six years, during which I'd been exposed to a quite phenomenal and broad amount of scientific information about the disease – and yet I still struggled to see how it all fitted together. During Hanahan's talk, in an over-warm, crowded Birmingham conference venue, I had a small professional epiphany – a flash of clarity, as all that information precipitated to form something ordered, comprehensible and structured. For the first time, I felt like I really understood the broad sweep of what researchers were learning about the biology of cancer. And so it seems sensible to use this framing to explain what – at around the time of Zarah's diagnosis – I understood about the disease.

Hanahan and Weinberg began their essay by pointing out that research had, so far, shown that the scrambled genes inside cancer cells seemed to be mutated in an almost infinite combination of ways, and that this was different from patient to patient – and even from cell to cell within a given patient. Frustratingly, despite decades of research, there appeared to be no 'master cancer genes', always faulty in every patient.

However, they observed, these myriad defects tended to cluster around a particular subset of biological processes – and these, they proposed, were the underlying hallmarks of the disease. Going further, they argued that cancers develop stepwise, collecting one hallmark after another, only becoming truly malignant after they've acquired the full set.

In some ways, this was nothing new – researchers had long worked out that cells need to accumulate a number of faults to become fully malignant. But Hanahan and Weinberg's 'hallmarks' provided a new pair of metaphorical spectacles through which to view cancer – one that I, personally, still find extremely useful when thinking about the disease. In particular, they emphasised an important point I made at the beginning of this section – that to form a full-blown growing, spreading tumour, cancer cells must subvert, and then collaborate with, their immediate surroundings.

The first of their hallmarks proposed that, unlike normal cells – which only multiply when they receive a 'green light' signal from their environment, explicitly telling them to do so – all cancer cells work out how to 'green light' themselves. In other words, they develop the ability to **keep growing in the absence of external signals**. Quite how they do this varies from cancer to cancer. Prostate cancer cells, for instance, frequently switch on genes that allow them to produce their own testosterone; other forms of cancer – such as breast cancer – can produce large quantities of hormone receptor proteins, allowing them to use low, ambient levels of hormone to keep growing. Other cancers, notably bowel and lung cancers, often overproduce the EGFR protein, or others like it.

But as well as these transient growth signals, cells also constantly receive messages from their neighbours telling them NOT to proliferate. And it seems that a cell needs both the presence of a 'go' signal and the absence of a 'stop' signal in order to divide. And so Hanahan and Weinberg's second hallmark – to stick with a traffic light analogy – is that all cancers must learn how to 'skip red lights' and **ignore signals from their surroundings that tell them not to divide**. Again, researchers have uncovered a whole suite of ways they can do this, such as deleting key sensor genes, or producing proteins that render them insensitive.

The first two hallmarks are relatively straightforward, but the third needs a little bit of context. In the 1970s, researchers discovered, buried deep within the human genome, a molecular suicide switch, able to trigger an ordered series of events leading to the complete breakdown of the cell. The researchers called the process triggered by this cellular death software 'apoptosis', a word derived from Ancient Greek for 'falling from' (*apo*, meaning 'from', and *ptosis*, meaning 'falling') and chosen because of the way, every autumn, trees divest themselves of their leaves in a tightly regulated manner. It's since turned out that apoptosis (the second 'p' is silent) is a vital part of how our bodies form and are regulated – and as well as causing worn-out, cancer-prone cells to self-destruct, it's also why you don't have webbed hands and feet but a newt does (it's apoptosis that breaks down this webbing in the embryos of developing mammals, but not in amphibians). Consequently, there are a variety of networks within a cell that can trigger apoptosis in different circumstances; Hanahan and Weinberg argued that, to become a cancer, cells must develop the ability to ignore them. Hence, their third hallmark is that all cancer cells are **resistant to apoptosis**.

To explain the fourth hallmark, I need to skip back to something I mentioned in passing earlier – the little shoelace-tip-like structures protecting the ends of chromosomes, called telomeres. As well as physically protecting our chromosomes from fraying, these have another, important property: they act as a tiny molecular clock – evolution's way of stopping our cells getting so worn out that they're likely to develop errors that could lead to cancer. Thus, in most of your cells, each time they divide, their telomeres get slightly shorter. When they're too short – after about 60 or so divisions – the cell is blocked from dividing any further (and often, at that point, triggers its apoptosis systems). Again, cancers often bypass this safety mechanism – either by switching on dormant systems that replenish and renew their telomeres, or by ignoring the signals sent out when they get too short. Either way, Hanahan and Weinberg proposed that all cancer cells effectively **become immortal**.

For the fifth hallmark, let's think again about the healing wound I discussed at the start of the section – and in particular, how the healing involves the growth of new blood vessels. This ability – which researchers have called 'angiogenesis' (from the Greek: *angio*, meaning 'vessel') – is encoded in our genes, tightly regulated and almost always switched off. But cancers consume vast amounts of energy to grow, and – consequently – need a constant supply of nutrients and oxygen. Hence, they need to somehow replumb their local blood supply, and to do this, they must somehow switch on angiogenesis pathways – either their own, or that in their surroundings. So Hanahan and Weinberg proposed that all cancers must **continuously grow new blood vessels**.

The next hallmark is, perhaps, the most obvious – if perhaps one of the least scientifically well understood. What makes cancers lethal is their ability to **invade into their surroundings and spread around the body** – a phenomenon called metastasis (yep, Greek again: 'remove' or 'change'). An oft-repeated (yet strangely hard to reference) statistic is that 90 per cent of cancer deaths are caused by the disease spreading to, and adversely affecting, other parts of the body. Quite how it does this is still hard to pin down, and researchers have found all sorts of mechanisms that cancers use to spread. Some seem to spread almost by accident – a growing tumour sheds its cells into nearby cavities, the blood or lymph systems, where they travel to other areas of the body and start growing. Others seem to physically burrow through tissues, activating genetic programs designed only for use in the cells of a growing embryo or a patrolling white blood cell. Much attention has turned in recent years to something called the 'seed and soil' hypothesis – the idea that cancers release signals into the bloodstream that somehow cause other organs and tissues to subtly change, becoming more hospitable to a growing cell. The different ways cancers do this explains, in part, why some types prefer to spread to the lungs, whereas others prefer the brain or liver. Either way, this sixth hallmark is a biggie – and as a result, understanding how cancer spreads is a critical focus of research. There is much still to learn.

Each of these six hallmarks describes an ability that a tumour acquires as it evolves. And so each must, on some level, result from a cell's DNA acquiring some sort of defect. But, Hanahan and Weinberg pointed out, in a normal cell, these sorts of errors are relatively rare, thanks to the presence of multiple error correction mechanisms – so rare, they pointed out, 'that the multiple mutations known to be present in tumor cell genomes are highly unlikely to occur within a human lifespan'. And yet, self-evidently, cancer still happens. There was obviously part of the picture missing. Thus, Hanahan and Weinberg also proposed a seventh hallmark, distinct from the other six, which they described as an 'enabling' hallmark: cancer cells must all have **highly unstable genomes**. 'We place this acquired characteristic of genomic instability apart from the [other hallmarks] – it represents the means that enables evolving populations of premalignant cells to reach [them],' they wrote.

These seven hallmarks – proposed in January 2000 – appeared to encompass everything then known about cancer. It was a remarkable achievement. The original Hallmarks essay came accompanied by a nifty diagram, which immediately began to crop up in PowerPoint presentations in lecture halls the world over. But of course, science is never fixed in time – new knowledge continually emerges, theories are constantly revised – and so, as Doug Hanahan told us in that conference

FIGURE 1 The Hallmarks of Cancer

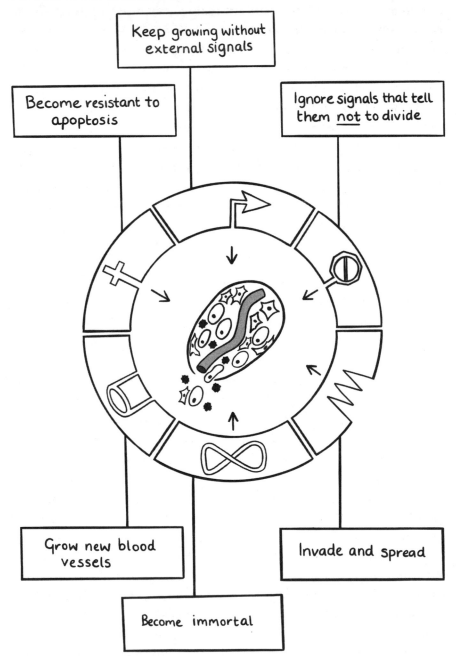

hall a decade later, he and Bob Weinberg had reviewed this evidence and proposed an additional three hallmarks, which they published in an updated essay called, with an almost Hollywood-like flourish, 'Hallmarks of Cancer: the Next Generation'.

The first drew on something I alluded to earlier – the fact that cancers consume vast quantities of energy in order to sustain themselves. To do this, researchers have learned, they need to ramp up their metabolism, using a variety of molecules from their immediate environment beyond glucose and fats. Thus, cancers are also characterised by a phenomenon called **deregulated energy metabolism**.

The second is a hugely important phenomenon we'll cover in more detail later on, so I won't dwell on it here, but it's cancer's ability to **evade the immune system** – something that's absolutely critical for it to be able to do simply to survive in the body. Understanding how it does this, and how to reverse it, has yielded some of the most exciting breakthroughs in cancer research – the advent of immunotherapies.

The final 'new' hallmark is – like having unstable genomes – another 'enabling' characteristic, and it harks back to my points earlier about a tumour being more than just cancer cells. They're made of all sorts of other 'normal' cells, co-opted to help sustain its growth, and this involves an extraordinarily complex crosstalk between the cancer cells and their neighbours. And the more researchers have learned to eavesdrop on this conversation, the more they've found it resembles a natural process, albeit one gone badly wrong: inflammation. When a tissue becomes damaged – as we saw with the example of wound healing earlier – a whole series of events kicks off, ultimately leading to the rapid, albeit tightly controlled, generation of new tissue to heal the wound. Many of these processes have echoes in the development of a cancer – particularly those driven by cells called fibroblasts, which help marshal the healing process. It turns out that tumours are often full of fibroblasts, responding to signals released by the cancer cells in a variety of inadvertent and unhelpful ways. Indeed, this – together with tumours' hallmark ability to grow new blood vessels by angiogenesis – has led to cancer being described as 'the wound that never heals'. There's now a sizeable body of evidence that chronic, long-term inflammation – caused, for example, by asbestos or certain infections – might actually be the starting point for a cancer's development, causing cells to multiply more rapidly, and making DNA errors more likely. So the final new hallmark proposed by Hanahan and Weinberg is **chronic, tumour-promoting inflammation**.

So there you have it. That's almost everything I knew about cancer by early 2016, when the disease so fatefully, personally, intervened in our lives, and Zarah was told she probably had cancer.

I'd like to be able to describe the conversations, the looks, the emotions that tumbled out during the next few weeks. In truth, it's a blur. There were so many unknowns and unknowables, we just got our heads down and got on with it, trying to keep everything as normal as we were able.

Obviously, we had to tell people. If anything, that's almost worse than being told. The uncomfortable silences. The shock. The reassurances that it will be OK. I clearly remember my dad's reaction – 'Oh, shit' – but I remember little else. I often wonder whether part of the myth around cancer, the taboo, comes in part from the shock the news instils in others outside the immediate bubble, as much as from the direct toll of the disease itself. Doctors are (usually) expert at imparting bad news; the rest of us less so. As conversation killers go, 'they think it's cancer' is hard to beat. Unlike the doctors, we'd had no training for this. It felt as if nothing in my decade at a cancer charity, talking about cancer every single day, was of use now.

Having reviewed the scans from Cork, the team at UCLH got in touch to say they'd managed to bring Zarah's appointment forward – could she come in today? At the time this felt hugely reassuring, but in retrospect was likely a sign that things were more urgent than we'd realised. Again, this is all a bit of a blur. We packed Zarah an overnight bag – the first of many over the coming months, the contents getting more honed, more useful and precise each time. Then we called a cab.

But we weren't heading to the main UCLH building – a huge, white, modern monolith – on London's busy Euston Road. Thanks to various reorganisations and restructures, UCLH's urology department is to be found elsewhere, in another, older, building up the road near Harley Street: Westmoreland Hospital, a grand old building constructed over a century ago, but recently refurbished. It was here that Zarah's operation was to take place.

Zarah checked in the day before. Her brightly lit, third-floor single room overlooked a pub – 'Well, at least we'll be able to sneak out for a pint easily,' she'd said. Priorities, always.

That evening, as she settled into her room and bed, I stood outside in the corridor, whispering into my phone so as not to disturb the sleeping patients. It was the first of many conversations I was to have with Professor Charlie Swanton that had nothing to do with 'work'.

I'd first met Charlie in 2012, while working on a feature about his work for the Cancer Research UK blog, to accompany a high-profile paper he was publishing (of which more later). We'd hit it off instantly and developed a mutual respect and rapport that several in my team (the cheeky sods) were wont to describe as a 'bromance'. Whatever the relationship had been up until then, it now took on a whole new dimension.

Charlie is a particular breed of doctor – a 'clinician scientist' – who interrupted his medical training to do a PhD in cancer research at the charity's London Research Institute, before resuming his medical career to become a fully fledged consultant oncologist (albeit one who has a deep knowledge of the biological processes affecting his patients). His passion for marrying scientific research with a clinical career comes, in part, from his frustration at the slow pace of research in bringing benefits to patients. 'I enjoyed medicine, but it was treading water,' he said in an interview in 2018. 'I didn't feel we were making progress.'[1]

Charlie's specialist subject – and that of his 30-strong research group – is how tumours evolve and adapt to treatment. His 2012 discovery, looking at this phenomenon in kidney cancer, had made headlines around the world, and he'd always been grateful for the role Cancer Research UK had played in both funding and popularising it. His team, now based jointly between UCLH and the then brand new Francis Crick Institute in King's Cross, were rapidly developing expertise in understanding how to 'read' cancer's faulty DNA to look for clues as to the rules governing how individual tumours grow and evolve – and, ultimately, how to treat the disease better.

I'd emailed him the previous night, just after midnight. 'Hey Charlie. I'm not sure how to begin this email, so I'm just going to go straight into it. My girlfriend Zarah is under investigation at UCLH for suspected bladder cancer. She's 37.'

I'd asked if, given the uniqueness of Zarah's case, his team would be interested in studying samples from her tumour, in case any information might prove useful to patients in the future. 'I know you get hundreds of requests like this, and I realise this might come across as a bit dispassionate (I'm sure you can imagine, the last 5 days have been anything but!)', I'd written. I didn't dare add that I hoped he might find some clues as to how to help Zarah – but, looking back, the unwritten implication screamed out from the email. A very British cry for help.

He'd replied at seven o'clock the following morning. From a research point of view there was little they'd be able to conclude, scientifically, from a single case. But he was desperate to help, and offered to try to find a way to collect and analyse tissue from Zarah's tumour to see if there were indeed any exploitable weaknesses, and copied in several team members to get the ball rolling. And also: 'If you want to talk, at any time, you know my number.'

It was like someone had thrown us a lifeline. Should this roller-coaster be heading off a cliff, if anyone on the planet could find a way to help us get off, or even just slow it down, I felt Charlie could.

Over the next 24 hours, I was copied into a series of frantic emails between various different clinicians as they arranged how to sort out the ethical approval and mechanics needed to get a sample of Zarah's bladder disease (it's worth saying that, at that point, we still didn't know for sure whether it actually was cancer).

So, that night, in the corridor of Westmoreland Hospital, Charlie and I caught up on the phone to check everything was in place for her operation tomorrow.

It was.

Phew.

'Henry, I'm so sorry this is happening,' he'd said.

Among the many tests Charlie's team planned to perform on Zarah's tumour sample, a crucial one was something called 'multi-region sequencing' – and to explain this jargony phrase, I need to break off for a minute and explain the nature of the genetic chaos inside cancer cells, and the role it plays in the disease's origin. It's going to get quite sciencey again, but don't worry – everything is relevant to Zarah's story. So let's pick up where we left off earlier – where I was talking about the scrambled, broken, error-riddled DNA inside cancer cells – and look at the story of how researchers have tried to map out and exploit these errors, with the ultimate goal of developing new ways to treat the disease.

A quick recap: one of the cancer cells' hallmarks is their unstable and disordered DNA, coiled up inside them and strewn with a whole catalogue of errors. Researchers now know, thanks again to decades of research on hundreds of thousands of patients' samples, that these errors can come in a variety of different types – often (in fact, usually) co-existing in the same cancer cell.

Some of these errors are tiny little 'spelling mistakes', where one or two 'letters' of a DNA sequence are missing, or substituted, or repeated. Researchers call these 'single nucleotide variants', or SNVs. They're probably the sort of thing you think of when you hear the word 'mutation' – actual changes to the order of rungs on the DNA ladder.

Others – called 'deletions' and 'amplifications' – involve (as you might expect) either the deletion of whole chunks of a particular chromosome's DNA or the repetition of other chunks, often many hundreds of times.

Yet more – dubbed 'fusions' or 'translocations' – can occur when entire chromosomes snap in two during cell division and are accidentally rejoined in the wrong order by the cell's inbuilt repair machinery.

And an even greater order of mistake can happen when entire chromosomes (and thus all the thousands of genes they bear) somehow get duplicated, and a cell contains multiple copies of them – a state known as 'aneuploidy', from the Greek: *an* meaning 'not', *eu* meaning 'good', and *plóos* meaning '-fold' (as in threefold).

So there are, we now know many types of genetic cancer chaos, from the tiny to the grotesque.

But regardless of whether they're tiny little SNV typos or gross aneuploid chromosome abnormalities (and leaving aside for now *how* they originate), all of these categories of error have one thing in common: they can alter a cell's behaviour by changing the information encoded in the genes inside the cancer cell.

Some SNV 'spelling mistakes' can lead to genes that produce proteins that are broken and inactive; others, conversely, can create permanently hyperactive versions. Or sometimes, they can cause the cell to make proteins that are *inappropriately* activated – bypassing the way they're normally controlled.

Similarly, duplicating whole chunks of DNA can mean a cell now contains multiple copies of a particular gene, again leading to its delicately balanced control systems going awry.

Continuing the theme, broken and rejoined chromosome 'fusions' can mean genes' usual control mechanisms – the little 'street signs' telling the cell how and when to activate them – become substituted for another's, again leading to inappropriate activity and loss of control. In fact, as we'll see below, in very rare cases the break points happen bang in the middle of two genes – splicing them back together in the wrong way can create new, hybrid genes that can cause the cell to do completely new things, a 'rare' situation that actually happens very frequently in a form of leukaemia.

And the duplication of entire chromosomes – aneuploidy – also upsets the delicate balance of control inside the cell, by duplicating all the genes on it. (See? I told you it all comes back to *control*.)

But as well as losing control of their behaviour, aneuploid cells also have another property – one that, as we'll see later, turned out to be extremely important in Zarah's case.

For a start, the extra chromosome(s) means there's a whole lot more DNA in each cell – more instructions that need to be faithfully copied each time they divide, more tangled spaghetti to pull apart, and a greater chance of something going wrong. And second, an aneuploid cell now has a 'spare' copy of each gene, which can go on to become mutated itself – and since that gene's original function is preserved on the original copy of the chromosome, a new mutated version can confer additional superpowers on the cell that contains it.

This means that the genetic information each cell contains is extremely unstable. As such cells divide, their progeny accumulate more errors, and, potentially, more 'superpowers' – such as resistance to cancer drugs, or the ability to spread around the body.

Over the years, as researchers learn more and more about these different types of DNA disruption and try to pin down their effects on cancer's development, a crucial concept has emerged. It turns out that, despite most cancers containing hundreds or thousands of mutations, only a small minority of the DNA changes in a given cancer cell directly cause its disordered growth. The rest seem to be 'collateral damage', accumulated as the cancer cells replicate their DNA every time they divide. Turning to an automobile-inspired analogy, these two categories of mutation have become known as 'driver' and 'passenger' mutations – the latter being merely 'along for the ride'. (To make things even more complex, the random nature of how different tumours originate means a particular gene fault can be the 'driver' of one person's cancer, but an accidental 'passenger' in another's. Context is everything, it seems.)

Now, in theory, if you can work out which gene or genes in a particular individual's cancer are the 'driver' genes, and how they help a tumour slip the shackles of normal control, you're on the way to working out how to guide it in a new direction: you can try to design drugs that are targeted to correct the effects of a particular gene fault – hence the name 'targeted' drugs. And over the last few decades, this incredibly simple idea has jump-started a huge research effort across academia and the pharmaceutical industry – an effort that has accelerated as researchers' ability to analyse the DNA inside cancer cells has improved apace. And it's yielded a host of new, weirdly named drugs that are either approved for routine use or working their way through clinical trials – some of which have already transformed how certain types of cancer are treated.

The story of one such targeted drug – imatinib – is regarded, in the field of cancer research, as its poster-child. And since it's literally a textbook story of how painstaking laboratory discoveries get translated directly into effective drugs, it's been beautifully covered in virtually every modern book about cancer. Even so, it's important context, so worth recapping here.

The story begins in Philadelphia, in the 1960s, where a team of researchers were studying a slow-burning form of leukaemia – chronic myelogenous leukaemia (CML for short). When they looked at DNA from patients' cancer cells down a microscope, they found that almost all of them contained a short, abnormal chromosome, which they dubbed the Philadelphia chromosome. This turned out to be a unique hallmark of the disease, found in almost every patient who develops it. But its precise role took another decade to decipher. In the 1970s, brand new lab techniques revealed that this stunted chunk of rogue DNA was formed early in the disease's course, when an ancestor of the leukaemia cells, struggling with a tricky bout of cell division, had tried to rejoin two broken chromosomes – chromosome 9 and chromosome 22 (a reminder from earlier: human cells contain 23 pairs of chromosomes), but accidentally joined them back the wrong way round. This genetic mix-and-match, which seems to be *the* fundamental cause of CML, has the unfortunate effect of joining a portion of a gene on chromosome 9, called '*abl*', to another gene on chromosome 22, called *BCR*. The resulting hybrid gene, known imaginatively as *BCR-abl*, bears corrupt instructions, telling the cell to make a mutant protein (also, imaginatively, called BCR-abl) that dramatically accelerates the rate at which it multiplies.

The discovery of the Philadelphia chromosome in the 1960s, followed in the 1970s by the hybrid gene it harboured, then allowed researchers to spend the 1980s working out how to isolate and purify the hyperactive BCR-abl protein from leukaemic patients' cells, and then test thousands of chemicals to try to find one that would switch it off again – and, hopefully, stop leukaemia cells from multiplying. By the late 1990s, they'd found one that could actually kill CML cells growing in a Petri dish with unique precision. Clinical trials began in 1998, and it was approved for routine use a few years later. It's sold under the name Gleevec, and by 2016 it was earning the drugs company Novartis more than $3bn worldwide.

More importantly, a follow-up trial of people taking the drug long-term, published in 2011 in the *Journal of the National Cancer Institute*,[2] showed that these patients **had normal life expectancies**. Before its discovery, they would all have had multiple rounds of chemotherapy, followed by a painful bone marrow stem cell transplant – often effective for some, but with brutal side effects. Most would have died. But by understanding the precise genetic fault inside these patients' cells, and its consequences, they could now take a pill for life, and hold their cancer at bay.

The development of imatinib appeared to be, as the cliché goes, a 'game changer', confirming the simple rules researchers thought they'd figured out: first, find the dodgy gene driving cancer cells' aberrant growth; then work out its effects; then develop a drug to counter them... and save lives. As I said earlier, it's perhaps the archetypal example of how cancer drug research is 'supposed' to work, and the excitement of translating these principles to generate more cancer drugs was, at that time, huge.

Except, as with everything in cancer, it was never going to be that simple. Of course it wasn't. The rules by which cancer plays would turn out to be vastly more complex.

Several other drugs appeared at around the same time, relying on similar principles. You may even have heard of some of them. Trastuzumab – better known by its commercial name, Herceptin – owes its existence to the discovery, in the 1980s, that breast tumours are often 'driven' by a particular gene amplification: cancer cells in the tumour contain hundreds of copies of a gene called *HER2* – a close relative of the *EGFR* gene we met earlier in the chapter.

Under normal circumstances, like *EGFR*, the *HER2* gene contains the information a cell needs to make a receptor protein called Her2 (don't worry about what these acronyms stand for – as with many gene and protein names, they're relics from the historical backstory of their discovery, and don't reveal much of relevance to our story). Like EGFR, these receptors act like little antennae, receiving signals from a cell's external environment and, when stimulated in this way, causing the cell to multiply.

Breast cancer cells carrying an amplified *HER2* gene coat themselves with masses of Her2 protein, making the cells exquisitely sensitive to growth signals. Trastuzumab was meticulously designed to slip over these extra Her2 antennae, covering them up and thus preventing them from passing on these growth signals. It was more laboratory science that made its way into the clinic: trials in patients proved conclusively that the drug could slow the growth of breast cancer, and it became routinely used to help people with the disease.

Another landmark targeted drug is vemurafenib (marketed as Zelboraf), designed to exploit the fact that about half of all melanoma skin cancers are driven by a single 'spelling mistake' in a gene called

BRAF, causing the gene to make a permanently 'switched on' protein, again causing them to proliferate rapidly.

Both of these drugs, and others like them, were designed only to be given to patients after analysing a sample of their tumour. If the genetic mistake was present, they'd get the drug; if it wasn't, they wouldn't. As a result, people with 'Her2-positive' breast cancer are now routinely given trastuzumab; similarly, people with *BRAF* V600E-positive melanoma are given vemurafenib or other similar drugs ('V600E' is shorthand that tells researchers the exact spelling mistake in the *BRAF* gene: it specifies a DNA error that causes the 600th amino acid in the BRAF protein to be substituted from one – valine (V) – to another, glutamic acid (E).

You might wonder why I'm talking about drugs for breast cancer and melanoma in a book that's essentially about bladder cancer. Hold that thought – it'll soon become clear.

With these drugs, and others like them, arriving in the clinic, the world of cancer medicine was said to be on the cusp of a new era of 'personalised' therapy. Soon, its proponents evangelised, all the relevant gene faults in cancer would be discovered, and companion drugs to counter their effects invented. All patients would need was to have a gene test carried out on their tumour upon diagnosis, and they could be prescribed the right drug to counter their tumour's mutation. Simple. In fact, it was predicted that trastuzumab – a 'breast cancer' drug – could in theory be used to treat *any* tumour that tests showed harboured the *HER2* amplification; similarly, trials were launched testing vemurafenib in other cancers where the *BRAF* mutation was present.

Progress towards this effort was fuelled by the arrival of a powerful new DNA analysis technology called 'next-generation' sequencing, allowing researchers to map all of the mutations in a patient's tumour in a matter of hours, rather than years, for a cost of mere thousands of dollars. (If you consider that the first ever whole-genome sequencing effort – the Human Genome Project – cost $2.7 billion and took several decades, you'll get a sense of the technological advance this represented.)

Armed with their new toys, cancer researchers and pharmaceutical companies began a global effort to catalogue all of the fundamental gene faults linked to the disease. They started to learn that, while certain faults were characteristic of particular types of cancer, they weren't exclusive to that disease. For example, the *BRAF* mutation, discovered thanks to its prevalence in melanoma, was also found to be present in bowel cancer, albeit less often. And, importantly for this story, the Her2 amplification discovered in breast cancer also cropped up in other cancer types – notably bladder cancer.

So the view of the different cancer types as distinct from each other began to break down. An organ-specific view of cancer started to give way to a genetic one.

But here's the catch I alluded to earlier, the big elephant in the room: for most patients, none of these drugs were anything like as effective as imatinib had been in chronic leukaemia. Sure, patients would often respond at first, sometimes dramatically... only to relapse later, often even more dramatically. This was particularly true of vemurafenib. I remember sitting in a conference hall in Liverpool in the late 2000s, as now iconic data from the early trials in melanoma were presented.[3] Three photographs appeared on the screen, side by side. On the far left, the patient before treatment, his pallid torso covered in golf-ball-like melanoma metastases. In the middle was a photo of what looked like a normal human torso, the golf balls banished, everything smooth and regular. It was miraculous. No drug had done anything like this for melanoma patients, ever.

And then on the right-hand side, the patient's torso several weeks later. The golf balls were back with a vengeance. They were everywhere. The drug worked for a while, but the cancer had found a way round. The patient died soon after. So near, and yet so far.

And, as well as the problem of drug resistance, another paradox was emerging. The trials of targeted drugs in cancers other than the cancer type they'd originally been developed to treat were often unsuccessful. Vemurafenib bombed in patients with bowel cancer bearing the *BRAF* V600E mutation.* Trastuzumab, while working reasonably well in a rare form of stomach cancer, had no effect in HER2-positive bladder cancer. By the late 2000s, optimism was starting to give way to a glum sense of cynicism. Why didn't these drugs work as well as imatinib? How were tumours becoming resistant to them? Why didn't they work as well in other cancers?

---

*However, laboratory scientists soon discovered why, and the drug is now used in combination with two other targeted drugs to treat certain forms of bowel cancer.

One of the underlying reasons began to be revealed, as researchers – notably, for our story, including Charlie Swanton's team – began looking at the precise cellular and genetic make-up of whole tumours, and, crucially, how this changed over time.

By the early 2000s, several labs around the world were trying to explain a critical observation: not all cancer cells in a patient's tumour were identical, a phenomenon called 'intratumour heterogeneity'. You can think of a tumour as being made of a patchwork of cells with slightly different mutations. It was a phenomenon first observed back in the 1970s, but crashed into the mainstream in 2012, when Charlie's lab published, in the *New England Journal of Medicine*, an analysis of the genetic make-up of a single patient's kidney cancer, in unprecedented detail.[4]

What set this study apart from hundreds of previous cancer gene studies was that, rather than analysing (or 'sequencing') the DNA genome from a single sample of the patient's kidney (as would be the case in a conventional gene test), Charlie's team had collected and analysed multiple samples – not just from the tumour in the patient's kidney, but also from the secondary cancers in their chest wall and lungs. They were then able to compare the mutated genes and chromosome abnormalities in each sample. And what they found confirmed what many had long suspected.

The patient's primary kidney tumour was a patchwork quilt of different types of cancer cell, all evolving from a common ancestor, but all subtly different, with different mutations in each. Moreover, each of the secondary metastatic cancers spreading around the patient's body was also genetically distinct – each appearing to arise from a different region of the primary tumour, but also accumulating more mutations, in addition to the original ones, along the way.

To make sense of this, the team developed sophisticated computer software that allowed them to crunch all this data, work out how 'related' each sample was to each other, and reconstruct the evolutionary history of the cancer's genetic abnormalities. Inspired by Darwin's famous 1837 'tree of life' sketch, the team represented this with a diagram – the original, early mutations in the cancer's history appear in the 'trunk' of the tree. And as different regions then evolve independently, the additional mutations are represented by 'branches'.

The technique that led to the metaphorical tree – the process of taking multiple samples from a patient, analysing them, and working out the 'driver' mutations in each – was dubbed 'multi-region sequencing'. And it had profound consequences for targeted, personalised cancer medicine.

To understand why, I want you to imagine something that may sound a little strange at first, but – please – bear with me. It's turkey time.

In the UK, it's generally called a three-bird roast, but in the US it's called a 'turducken'. It's a peculiarly ostentatious form of festive meal, whereby the chef inserts a chicken into a duck, and then the resulting, er, 'ducken' into a turkey.

There are also variants such as (in America) the gooducken (a chicken in a duck in a goose), Waitrose's popular four-bird roast (a guinea fowl in a duck in a turkey in a goose) and Hugh Fearnley-Whittingstall's frankly ridiculous ten-bird roast – an 18lb turkey with a goose, a duck, a mallard, a guinea fowl, a chicken, a pheasant, a partridge, a pigeon and a woodcock inside it. I don't know why.

(Stay with me, I know it's getting a bit off-piste.)

Now, imagine you've got a large, nondescript roast bird on the table in front of you, but you want to know what it is – a gooducken? a three-bird roast? just a turkey? – but all you've got to help you find out is a biopsy needle and a DNA sequencer. (Look, I didn't say this was going to be a realistic, everyday situation.)

You take one single sample, run it through the DNA sequencer, and the result says 'turkey DNA'. So, it's not the gooducken. But which of the other gastronomic monstrosities is it? Of course, you can't say for sure. You obviously need to take more than one sample. And the more samples you take, the more certain you are of what you're about to serve your guests.

Now let's get back to cancer (sorry, you're probably hungry now – or queasy). You can see the problem: if tumours are inherently variegated – if they contain many different regions, each with different mutations in them – a single tissue biopsy might well miss the true nature of the beast. Charlie's kidney cancer study – and a slew of others that followed quickly in its wake – strongly suggested that, to fully identify the genes driving a patient's tumour (and hence, which treatments to prescribe), more than one tissue biopsy should be taken – something that wasn't yet (and largely still isn't) being offered routinely.

The discovery of tumours' heterogeneous, variegated nature had another implication too: it offered a crucial reason why resistance almost inevitably developed, both to targeted drugs and to conventional chemotherapy. Cancers are made up of different regions (scientifically called 'clones') of cells, with differing levels of sensitivity to different drugs. Thus, drugs might wipe out one or more of these clones, but the remainder could – and invariably would – grow back.

Here's an example. Consider a patient being treated for advanced melanoma skin cancer. A biopsy is taken and analysed, and found to have the *BRAF* V600E mutation. In theory, the disease should be sensitive to vemurafenib. The patient is prescribed the drug...

... which does nothing. The doctors scratch their heads (and probably reach for the immunotherapy, but we'll get to that later). What the doctors didn't know – what the results didn't tell them – was that they'd taken a biopsy from a region of the patient's melanoma that had only acquired the BRAF mutation later on in the tumour's development. It was a passenger, not a driver. It was in a branch, not a trunk.* The melanoma wasn't a turkey, it was a turducken – and the chicken was in charge (I'm not sure that works, but hey).

So, now, armed with this understanding of the importance of the patchwork nature of tumours, let's get back to Zarah, asleep in Westmoreland Hospital, waiting for the mass in her bladder to be removed. What Charlie was offering to do – as a favour – was to take multiple samples from the resulting tissue, perform multi-region sequencing on it, and try to find out what mutations were driving her cancer.

It was an incredible, generous thing to do. And that's why, despite our predicament, I felt so hopeful. It meant that, should Zarah's tumour carry one of a handful of particular weaknesses, should that weakness be in the tumour's metaphorical 'trunk', and should we be able to (somehow) get hold of drugs to target it, then... It was a long shot – one in a million. But then she was one in a million herself.

---

*In practice, in melanoma, BRAF mutations are almost always in the 'trunk' of a tumour. Resistance to vemurafenib – which happens frequently – is instead because the tumour carries or develops other mutations that allow it to escape the drug's effects. But the basic principle here – that you can't know from a single biopsy sample whether a mutation is in a 'trunk' or a 'branch' – holds true.

Back in 2012, when I was writing the blog post to help publicise Charlie's kidney cancer discovery, when my team were working on the graphics that several newspapers adapted to spread the finding far and wide, when I sat in Charlie's London office and pestered him to explain it all *one more time* – I never for a moment suspected that the techniques he was describing, that I was scribbling down, that we were illustrating for the mass media would, four years later, be employed desperately to try to save my girlfriend's life.

The operation was going to take a few hours. I went down with her to the pre-op waiting area. We sat alone in a dimly lit room, waiting nervously for the call. The room was empty save for a solitary lifestyle magazine. 'Ten ways to a healthier body', that type of thing. I didn't check, but I'm pretty sure transurethral biopsies weren't on the list.

The call came, a kiss, a hand-squeeze. See you in a bit. So casual.

Upstairs, back in the waiting room, as Zarah presumably lay conked out on the operating table a few floors below, and as a researcher hovered at the end of the bed, waiting to whisk a sample of her tumour off to be analysed, I gazed into the distance and wondered what Charlie would find.

And, as I waited, I got my first glimpse of the altruistic chaos that is the modern NHS. A busy nurse popped her head in. 'Does anyone want tea or coffee?' she asked. She received a volley of complaints in reply. 'I've been waiting for ages, when will I get a bed?' 'Is he out yet, it's been three hours and no one will tell me anything'. I guiltily asked for a coffee: milk, no sugar. Well, she *had* asked. The nurse, her head now full of a million requests, disappeared off to try to make everyone's life better.

I earwigged on a conversation – the elderly couple opposite had travelled down from Leeds for specialist urology care, but had been bumped down the list and the operation would be tomorrow. There was no bed. They'd have to get a hotel. They were upset, furious. It later occurred to me who was being treated in their place. I felt not one shred of guilt.

The nurse eventually returned, full of information as requested. Not everyone was happy, but at least they were better informed. She turned to me, and a look of horror spread across her face. 'Oh God, I'm so sorry! I forgot your coffee.' Before I could stop her, she dashed off, to return a few moments later with a cup of instant. I'll likely say this repeatedly over the following pages, but these people are fucking heroes.

A groggy and disoriented Zarah was wheeled back up on a standard-issue NHS movable bed a few hours later – I arrived at her room at about the same time. I can't remember what we talked about for the rest of that evening; we were just relieved everything had gone according to plan, that whatever was in Zarah's bladder had been dispatched, and that Charlie had his samples.

V: The probe

Like a malign pink sea anemone, the alien mass extends out into the bladder, almost filling it.

Composed of billions of cells, this variegated monster has been slowly growing for years, fuelled by an anarchic network of blood vessels, bringing it vital oxygen and nutrients. It has now expanded and invaded aggressively in every direction – not just upwards and outwards, but downwards into the layer of muscle surrounding the bladder and beyond.

Each of its multitude of cells bears echoes of its past – the grotesquely disordered DNA, the deleted control switch, the hyperactive guardian, the amplified antenna gene – but entire lineages have acquired additional superpowers: distinct mutant families of cells, all distant grandchildren of the mother cell whose fateful error set this chain of events into motion.

While the early seeds of the monster's emergence were sown by catastrophe, fate and error, much of its subsequent pathological diversity, arisen in the intervening years, has had a different, self-inflicted source: evolution's own antivirus software – a molecular DNA cutter, able to precisely sense, and then scramble, the DNA of invading viruses.

Initially, its activation had been triggered in error by the slowly building chaos in the cells' nuclei, tricking these antiviral DNA scramblers into targeting the cells' own DNA, hard-coding mistake after mistake into the cells' genomes. But as the chaos built, the bladder's local immune cells, half-sensing a problem – slowly, lethargically – had attempted to heal the perceived insult, desperately pumping out chemical signals to summon help. But as well as calling in reinforcements, these signals had inadvertently boosted the monster's aberrant virus protection, wreaking wave after wave of damage on billions upon billions of already mangled genomes.

Although new mutant cells were constantly created, most had self-destructed, too damaged to go on. Others were spotted and eliminated by local immune cells, suddenly able to detect the presence of new, rogue, misshapen proteins on their surface. But the fittest survived and multiplied, allowing the monster to gain new abilities, and expand in new directions.

In parallel, over the same period, local immune cells' chatter gradually changed. Where once their signals cried 'help', over time – perhaps tricked by signals emitted by the monster itself, perhaps mis-sensing the chronic, smouldering monster as the final stages of a long-healing wound – they began to summon calming, regulatory macrophages to dampen down the low-level assault.

And so, the monster's growth continued unhindered, all shackles of control finally slipped.

But today, this complete dominance of its environment is about to change.

Gently, slowly, a thin metal probe enters the bladder and approaches the alien mass, at its tip a tiny loop of wire.

As the probe nears the surface of the mass, the wire glows red-hot. It presses against the monster, slicing again and again through the rogue tissue, cauterising broken and burst blood vessels as it does so. Smoke from the burnt, dead tissue fills the bladder.

Over and over, with brutal accuracy, the probe's wire burns through the mass, pruning it back to the surface of the bladder, slice by slice, until at last, barely any of its pathological bulk remains.

The next morning, The Surgeon entered the room. In keeping with that profession's stereotype, his bedside manner was brusque, dispassionate and businesslike – a walking, talking, cancer-removing cliché. His hands folded behind his back, staring out the window, he delivered the news. It hit us like a shell.

'Well, we got most of it out. But it's quite extensive. You'll need a nephrostomy – we'll book that in for tomorrow or the day after.'

The tumour, he told us, had gone through the muscular wall of the bladder and started to grow into the inner wall of Zarah's pelvis.

We were speechless. In the absence of any other information, we'd assumed that the operation would rid Zarah's bladder of the whatever-it-was. What The Surgeon was saying was, it was worse than we'd feared.

The form of bladder cancer that it was becoming clear Zarah likely had is known as 'muscle-invasive' bladder cancer. It starts among the cells that line the inside of the bladder, but then grows through the surrounding muscle and out into the abdominal cavity, then on towards the lymph nodes. Once it's grown this far, precise removal is impossible. The only way to get rid of it is an intensive, heavy-duty operation to remove the entire bladder, called a radical cystectomy – UCLH's expertise in this was one of the reasons it had been suggested for us. But the operation is pretty pointless, not to say risky, if the cancer has already spread beyond the bladder's confines.

The fact that a cystectomy hadn't been raised as an option was terrible news. The cancer – this, now, was definitely cancer – was very advanced.

The other kicker was that Zarah would need a nephrostomy – a tube drilled in through her back into her kidney, allowing urine to drain into a bag strapped to her leg. It is to wee what a colostomy is to poo. That Zarah would need one meant they hadn't been able to remove enough of the mass to get her swollen, blocked kidney working again.

The final, inevitable, implication of all this was the word we'd been dreading: chemotherapy.

After he left, Zarah's anger, miraculously absent till this point, flared up tearfully. 'He didn't even look me in the eye!'

Eventually, she drifted off to sleep, and I began the first of many, many late-night lonely journeys back to our empty flat. We were having work done on the kitchen, new worktops and appliances – suddenly so mundane. As I opened the door, unexpectedly I could hear music playing: the builders had left their plaster-coated radio on, stuffed in a corner, out of reach, behind our old, displaced washing machine.

It was playing Eric Carmen's 'All By Myself'.

I launched myself over the washing machine, legs in the air, frantically groping for the off switch.

The chorus echoed around the flat.

I stretched, found the switch, silenced the bloody thing. But the song continued to churn round my head. I sat in the middle of the kitchen floor and wept.

There were to be a couple more nights in Westmoreland before Zarah could come home. Each morning I'd get the Tube across London to the hospital.

On the second morning, I stopped at Tesco to pick up some supplies for Zarah, and grabbed a coffee for myself from the machine in the middle of the store – it was one of those set-ups where you make the coffee, then take it to the checkout to pay. But the card machine wasn't working, and I had no cash. 'Sorry. You'll have to leave it here. But there's a cashpoint round the corner.' Bastard! I needed to get to the hospital urgently, I almost yelled, starting to lose it. Cashier said no. Then the woman behind me tapped me on the shoulder and offered to pay. I immediately dissolved in a flood of tears, again. This established another new, unanticipated fact about cancer, one that would recur again and again over the coming months: emotionally speaking, it's the kindness, more than the disease, that really gets you.

At the hospital, as I sipped a grotty, tasteless latte, we discussed the future: once a glowing, happy place, with a garden, a dog, some micro-pigs, a recording studio in the spare room, more travelling; now a surreal, cloudy, uncertain, risky place. We'd get there though. We would, we would.

Zarah had her nephrostomy a day later, under sedation rather than general anaesthetic. They had to give her an extra-large dose of sedative – she did have the constitution of an ox. Friends came to visit. Zarah charmed the nurses. Our spirits were strangely high as the two of us slowly absorbed the new reality, the new normal. Team Twat would do this together.

Eventually, we got the nod. We packed up, called a cab, and arrived back, relieved, exhausted: happy to be home. The new kitchen looked amazing.

A few days later, we were back at Westmoreland, to meet the consultant, to find out, finally, definitely, definitively, what type of cancer was growing in Zarah's bladder, how advanced it was, and what treatment would follow.

There were several possibilities: most of them bad, but some absolutely awful. Aside from the bog-standard, muscle-invasive form, there were other, weirder, rarer forms. These had less definite treatments, and were (according to my late-night forays into Google) Pretty Fucking Horrendous.

We sat in the waiting room on the ground floor, a typical bright, strip-lit soulless enclosure with doors on every wall, each bearing the hastily scribbled name of whichever NHS employee was currently operating out of it. We were to see Dr Mark Linch – I recognised his name from the emails Charlie Swanton had sent out previously.

Mark opened the door and called us in. He's a lovely man, is Mark: not far off our age, personable, kind, approachable – and he rapidly became one of our favourites. He was so good with Zarah, the epitome of 'caring and compassionate'. We sat down. Mark started speaking. I remember the information, but barely the actual words.

Zarah, Mark said, had muscle-invasive, transitional cell bladder cancer – the 'bog-standard', most common type. It was 'high grade', meaning, on the one hand, fast-growing and aggressive; on the other, more often sensitive to chemotherapy. And then came the phrase we'd been steeling ourselves for, dreading.

'It's stage 4.'

There are only four stages; stage 4 is, for most types of cancer, when the disease has spread to an extent that it can't usually be cured with surgery, radiotherapy or chemotherapy.

Chemo could, however, drastically hobble the disease, stopping it in its tracks, and buying us time. We didn't dare ask how much – averages aren't much help. I do remember Mark advising us not to focus on the statistics – Zarah was young, fit, healthy; the fact that she had cancer so young meant it was unlikely to be a 'typical' cancer.

There were other, tiny straws of consolation, which we eagerly grasped at. Although the cancer had spread to the lymph nodes adjacent to Zarah's bladder, there was no sign of the disease in either her lungs or liver – the next stops on bladder cancer's inevitable journey. (So with a good wind, we could be looking at years, I remember thinking, but not saying.)

Ashen-faced, shaking, we left, Mark's eyes full of sadness too. As I walked out the door, he put his hand on my shoulder. 'I'm really sorry.' I wanted to hug him – this kindly man I'd only just met, who'd given us this awful, awful news.

As we left the hospital, we didn't know what to do with ourselves. 'Fancy a coffee?' 'Why not.' Several doors down from Westmoreland is a typical trendy coffee shop, the kind with stupidly uncomfortable but stylish seating and overpriced lattes.

I can't remember what we talked about. But I can remember clearly it being the worst, most tasteless, most awfully sad coffee I've ever drunk.

And as we waited for a cab, I can remember holding Zarah's hand tight, watching her ever-present eyeliner run gently down her pale, beautiful cheek.

3

Chemotherapy

FUCK CANCER. LET'S GO to the cinema. We walked from our flat down Cambridge Heath Road to Whitechapel. Or maybe we got the bus. I can't remember, it just felt so good to be out, to be normal, to be walking down the road holding hands, to see a film, as if nothing had ever happened, as if we weren't carrying this weight, this fate. The normality made us feel temporarily invincible. Zarah was still in pain from the operation, slightly encumbered by the nephrostomy bag on her leg. But as if that was going to stop her. As if it would ever stop her.

We passed the big Sainsbury's supermarket in Whitechapel. It was – still is – clad in temporary facades and scaffolding, as much construction site as supermarket, due to the imminent subterranean arrival of a new Crossrail station. As Wikipedia will tell you, Crossrail is 'a 118-kilometre (73-mile) railway line under development in England, running through parts of London and the home counties of Berkshire, Buckinghamshire and Essex'.

We'd been pretty excited about it; it aimed to link up several bits of London between which we frequently travelled – most notably, in Zarah's case, Whitechapel and Marks & Spencer's offices near Paddington. It would shave a good half-hour off her journey to work, the sort of thing that would in other circumstances be life-changing. It would probably do pretty decent things for the value of my flat, too.

Simultaneously, unthinkingly, we gazed up at the hoarding that loudly proclaimed the station's opening date in block caps:

'SUMMER 2018'.

As we looked back to the road ahead, I felt Zarah's hand tighten in mine. A tiny, almost imperceptible shudder. My vision blurred with moisture. We kept walking. I don't think we said anything, but we didn't need to.

We got to the cinema, the Genesis – a lovely independent former East End theatre, bought and resurrected by a son for his dad: the place where father courted mother four decades earlier. Chaplin, Laurel and Hardy had performed there, a place steeped in love, history and remembrance. And for once in our lives, we were early. Early enough for a large glass of red wine, which we drank with almost religious reverence – our first drink since we'd got the devastating news – gazing at each other across the table in the bar, eyes ablaze with relief and love, the earlier brief but crushing sadness driven away by our determination to be fucking normal and fucking drunk and not let this fucking disease ruin things.

The sheer raw joy of that memory sticks out, I don't know why – perhaps the counterpoints and contradictions of doing something so mundane in the face of what we'd just been through, and what was still to come. The film was brilliant – *The Big Short*, based on a true story, an exposé of the events leading up to the 2008 financial crash, when the world was turned upside-down and nothing was ever the same again.

It's amazing how many profound, world-changing events can be crammed into a single, short lifetime, isn't it?

'Oh God, will she lose her hair?' said my mum, on the phone, when I told her. It was the first question Zarah had had, too. It's the first thing everyone thinks of.

Chemotherapy. It's a fearful word. It literally means something mundane: 'medical treatment involving chemicals' – technically, every time you take a paracetamol, or an aspirin, that's chemotherapy. Of course, that's not what it *actually* means. Ask a random member of the public to write down or draw what images spring to mind, you'd likely get an anxiety-inducing list that includes concepts like 'baldness', 'painful', 'drip' and 'nausea'. Because, of course, in the public consciousness, chemotherapy is inextricably linked to the word 'cancer', and to ghastly media images of pallid, sick patients – often children – in hospital beds, or 'bravely' wandering around with whacky headscarves. It's a word with almost entirely negative connotations. A friend's mum, after treatment for breast cancer, had once told me, 'Henry, if your lot can do anything, for God's sake make the chemo less awful.'

Zarah's chemotherapy – an 18-week course of two different drugs, cisplatin and gemcitabine – was scheduled to start that Wednesday, barely a week after her operation, and just over a fortnight since we'd flown back from Ireland. I'll talk in more detail about these drugs later – how they work, where they come from, and why they (rather than any of the other scores of chemotherapy drugs in the pharmacist's armoury) are used to treat bladder cancer. For now, the following facts are all you need:

The drugs would be given one after another, intravenously, over a two-hour period. This would happen once a week for two weeks, then there'd be a week's break to let Zarah's system recover. This 'two weeks on, one week off' arrangement was to constitute one 'cycle' – there would be six cycles in total. Alongside this, for a few days after the chemo infusion, Zarah would take a couple of other drugs, as tablets, twice a day, to counteract any side effects that might arise: a steroid called dexamethasone, and a second anti-nausea drug called domperidone, which Zarah – and I suspect many others – ironically called 'Dom Perignon'.

All of this would be given to her as an outpatient, on Wednesday afternoons. We could both go back to work, and try to regain a semblance of normality.

At least, that was the plan. But the First Rule of Cancer, we rapidly learned, is: fuck your plans.

That Monday night, two days prior to Chemo Round 1, the pain in Zarah's abdomen suddenly sharpened. She threw up. Her temperature spiked. At dawn, with no improvement in sight, we phoned the UCLH cancer patient hotline; they said, 'Go straight to A&E' (they may as well have added, 'Do not pass Go, do not collect £200').

UCLH is one of the best hospitals in the UK. It's also one of the busiest. A trip to its hectic A&E department, therefore, wasn't something to be undertaken lightly. As I helped pack her overnight bag, I feared the worst – Zarah was in quite a bad way, and the prospect of several hours among Central London's drunk, vomiting and broken wasn't terribly appealing.

I needn't have worried: if you're a cancer patient with a temperature, you can generally jump at least the first bit of the queue (which at any rate, at 7 a.m., was pretty sparse), and Zarah was quickly found a cubicle and hooked up to a drip of antibiotics and morphine by a surprisingly cheerful nurse. The morphine was an absolute godsend – for the first time in more than a month, she was suddenly, mercifully, joyously pain-free. In the small, brightly lit cubicle, separated from the chaos by a mere curtain, she gave out a hugely contented, relieved sigh, and went straight to sleep.

The cause of this little episode was revealed later that day – Zarah had a nasty bladder infection, and this would mean postponing the first round of chemo until it had cleared (chemo squashes the immune system – it's not a good idea to give it to someone with an active infection). The rest of the day was spent waiting for a ward bed to become available, and at about eight o'clock that evening she was eventually transferred, for the very first time, up to the inpatients' ward on floor 14 of the hospital's main tower. It's a modern, clean, busy ward – so busy that should you pop out for coffee, or supplies, you often have to wait outside, pressing the buzzer over and over, before a nurse or kindly visiting family member will let you in.

That first night, due to her infection, Zarah got a private room, with a little fridge, a separate bathroom, and a glorious view of London's skyline. In any other circumstances, this sort of accommodation would be well out of our price range. Cancer has some benefits, I guess.

The following day, at Zarah's bedside, we had our first proper meeting with her consultant oncologist: Dr Ursula McGovern.

We'd met Ursula once before, very briefly, when Zarah was over at the urology department in Westmoreland – she'd popped round to introduce herself, shortly after we'd got the news from the surgeon that he hadn't been able to remove all of the cancer. A kind, friendly, slightly maternal woman, we'd warmed to her then, particularly after the brusque demeanour of the surgeon. She had Irish roots, and she and Zarah had quickly dropped into chat about where in Ireland her family were from.

Now she was here to talk more fully about the chemo Zarah would have, to explain the plan to deal with the current infection, and answer any questions we might have. Again, I don't remember much about the specifics of the conversation – over the course of her illness, we'd have so many bedside conversations with so many different doctors – but my overriding memory of our first encounter with Ursula was of someone deeply caring, incredibly reassuring, but also desperate to keep our feet on the ground, not over-promise anything, and not get drawn into thinking too far ahead. I think this may have been where I first enquired about the possibility of immunotherapy – 'We need to try what we know works first' was the gist of the answer. That's a sentence, a sentiment, that's run round and round my head ever since.

In the short term, the plan was simple. The chemo planned for Wednesday would be postponed, and they'd keep Zarah in until her infection cleared up – if it was gone before the weekend, they'd give her chemo on the ward, and then discharge her, and the second dose of Round 1 could then go ahead next week. We'd be on schedule. But if the infection took longer, they'd push things back to the following week, and everything would take place a week later.

This worried us for two reasons. First, the obvious one: we were both keen to get cracking, to start pouring toxic chemicals into Zarah's veins and try to buy as much time as we could, sod the side effects, sod the consequences. We were quickly reassured about the delay – a week was, in the grand scheme of things, neither here nor there, and wouldn't make a difference clinically to the overall picture. But second, we had various holidays and trips booked that we were desperate not to miss out on. In retrospect, now knowing how cancer forces you to suspend everything, puts your whole life on hold, becomes your master, your diary planner, your overlord, this seems totally naive. But at the time, it seemed a rational thing to worry about. The main thing on the horizon was my Christmas present: Zarah had bought us flights to Ljubljana in Slovenia, and in early January, before all this, we'd spent a lazy morning in bed looking at beautiful, cosy little apartments on Airbnb, and were both really excited to go – even more so now. The flights she'd booked fell, by coincidence, right in the week off between the first and second of the planned chemo cycles. Changing them, or cancelling them, was an extra ball to juggle, a hassle we did not need.

Later that day, Zarah's temperature began to fall as the antibiotics kicked in. While this was good news in the long run, it meant giving up the private room and moving to the main ward, to a four-person arrangement with mere curtains for privacy. The other three patients were all very elderly, with advanced disease, and in a terrible way – hacking, wheezing, moaning uncontrollably. It was a horrible set-up – Zarah's very first night on an oncology ward proper offered an unpalatable glimpse into a possible future that knocked her sideways, psychologically. The next day I had a quiet, hopeful word with a nurse – Zarah was young and newly diagnosed, this wasn't a good place for her, were there any other options? Thankfully, the other end of the ward was for younger patients, and a bed had just become available; we were swiftly moved. Like I said, heroes.

So Zarah's third night was much more comfortable, less distressing. And on the Friday morning, her blood test results came back OK: the infection was gone, chemo could go ahead. We were on schedule. Phew.

It was just before this that I sent out the first of what would become a series of long, involved emails to our family and friends, to keep them in the loop about what was going on, and to explain what was happening and why. That afternoon, I sent a short update that just reads, 'Chemo going ahead in a couple of hours. Yay, of sorts.'

For such a fearful concept, the reality of having chemotherapy is rather mundane, and I was mildly shocked by the realisation that despite nearly 14 years writing about cancer, I'd never actually 'seen' chemotherapy in the wild. Here's how it worked. Zarah had been on a saline drip for much of her time on the ward – a clear bag of liquid suspended from a pole, with a tube going via an electric pump into a cannula in her left arm. For all the dramas, anxiety and anticipation, 'having chemotherapy' – this brutal, life-extending elixir – involved two nurses wheeling over another bag of clear liquid, asking Zarah her date of birth, swapping the new bag for the nearly-empty saline bag, pressing a few buttons on the front of the pump, then wandering off again.

The first bag – the cisplatin – took an hour to infuse. Then it was swapped over with a smaller bag of similarly clear liquid – the gemcitabine – for another half an hour. Then another half-hour bag of saline, just to make sure she was properly hydrated. Zarah was given a couple of tablets of dexamethasone and domperidone to keep any nausea at bay, then it was time to pack up and go home. It was a huge, if welcome, anticlimax. While we waited for Zarah to be formally discharged, the steroids kicked in and she became ravenously hungry. So the first observable side effect of chemotherapy I ever saw was Zarah wolfing down a slightly dry NHS-issue cheese sandwich.

A quick note about the process of being discharged from hospital. It's invariably, predictably, chaotically shit. You can be left hanging for ages: you're not supposed to go without receiving a bunch of drugs and a formal discharge letter. The former can take literally hours to arrive – more so on busy times, such as Friday nights, or times of short-staffing, like weekends. Over the time Zarah was ill, I reckon we lost the best part of three or four whole days in total waiting for the pharmacy to sort their shit out. Sometimes the wrong drugs would arrive and have to be sent back; other times they'd apparently be given to a porter, who would go AWOL for hours on end. There are many frustrations with the current NHS set-up, but being discharged from hospital was, for us anyway, one of the absolute worst. And there's a flip side to it too, at the other end of the process – we'd also end up spending hours in A&E waiting for a bed to become available up in a ward, presumably while someone else, upstairs somewhere, was sitting, fully clothed, bags packed, waiting expectantly and desperately for the fucking pharmacy to sort out their prescription so they could go home. So next time you read about 'cutting back-room bureaucracy' in the NHS, this is the ultimate effect.

Anyway, eventually we got the drugs – a plastic goody bag containing boxes of slow-release morphine tablets, paracetamol, Oramorph (a liquid form of morphine for occasional 'breakthrough' pain), domperidone, dexamethasone, and some diazepam to help her sleep – called a cab, and headed back to the flat to hunker down and see what this chemotherapy shit was all about.

VI: Chemical warfare

It has been days since the glowing probe's sustained assault, and the battered, bleeding monster is a remnant of its former self.

Where once it was a seething mass of billions of cells, now it is mere millions – a thin layer of disordered tissue penetrating into the surface of the bladder.

Within this thin stratum of tissue, the mother cell's diminished progeny continue to multiply and proliferate anew, trying to build back their number, diversifying once more as they do.

But not for much longer.

Slowly at first, but growing in intensity, seeping in through the bladder's capillaries and into the monster's own disordered supply, a new offensive begins. Chemical warfare on a cellular level.

Diffusing into each and every cell in the bladder: tiny primitive cross-shaped molecular complexes, each constructed around a highly charged metallic core, able to stick indiscriminately to the cells' intricate biomolecular contents.

Most lethally, the complexes bind to the abnormal, error-strewn DNA double helices wound tightly in the cells' nuclei, distorting them, fusing together the rungs of their chaotic ladders. The cells of the monster, dividing rapidly, are exquisitely vulnerable, their DNA exposed repeatedly as they try to multiply amid this toxic milieu.

Simultaneously, the complexes react with other components within each cell, stripping them of electrons, disintegrating them as they do, generating a cascade of smaller, charged atoms and molecules – each free to diffuse around the cell, causing more havoc.

Driven to divide, but sensing the catastrophic internal damage, cell after cell is pushed over the edge, triggering ancient self-destruct mechanisms, dissolving into a soup of biomolecules. Gradually, these remnants diffuse out into the surrounding tissue, attracting the attention of the immune system once more.

Other cells are also targeted by this cellular chemical warfare: the calming, immune-dampening macrophages that have long penetrated the monster's bulk, protecting it against onslaught. They, too, self-destruct in the toxic metal's presence, and as they do, their suppressive signals dissipate. For the first time since the monster's arrival, at last the bladder's immune system is free to attack – and it does so with lethal force.

Thus, the monster's remnants come under dual assault: internally from the toxic effects of the poison, and externally from the rejuvenated, unleashed power of the immune system.

An epic cellular battle for survival has begun.

Back in the safety of our flat, the weekend came and went, with little incident save, oh, a few hours on Saturday night where, full of steroids to offset the chemo's side effects, Zarah became convinced she was swelling up, so had me measure the circumference of her abdomen every few hours – she wasn't swelling up, it was 'just' the steroids making her a bit paranoid. The steroids basically added '...on steroids' to any emotion she felt. The flat got tidied. Twice. So much for fatigue. The knackered one was me, dealing with a hyperactive girlfriend.

Zarah's nervous steroidal energy found an incredibly useful outlet in the form of flower arranging – because, bless 'em, every Tom, Dick and Harriet had also decided to send us flowers. As I wrote in an email at the time, 'Seriously, there should be something on the Cancer Research UK website to warn you that, if you ever get cancer, you immediately need to buy at least six new vases and a magazine rack.' Sarcasm aside, the response from everyone was overwhelmingly lovely. As I said earlier, the kindness is the stuff that really gets you – each new package induced floods of grateful tears from both of us. It wasn't just flowers – lip balm, colouring books, cashmere jumpers, vouchers, everything. Amazing.

But anyway, we were all aboard the good ship chemotherapy – which had, miraculously, departed only slightly late, and was still on schedule for its next stop. Right? Ha. No. Not a minute of it. It's cancer. You don't get to relax. You never get to relax. Keep your eyes on the horizon, the waters are pretty fucking choppy.

We both went back to work on Monday and Tuesday. Normality – you cling to the normality. Then, on Wednesday, as planned, we headed into UCLH for the second dose of chemo. Zarah by this time was starting to feel a bit woozy and feverish – something we naively ascribed to the chemo. Oopsy.

The UCH Macmillan Cancer Centre is set a few streets away from UCLH proper. It's a large, bright, airy, purpose-built block, with its own scanners and services, all tailored for people with cancer, taking the load off the main hospital's facilities. It's got a heavily branded green-and-white Macmillan information centre, full of lovely staff and well-written leaflets covering every possible aspect of the disease – 'SEX WHEN YOU HAVE CANCER' (no thanks, it's a bit public in here). It's a brilliant place in so many ways... but it has one glaring design flaw, which completely tripped us up on our first visit.

As you enter the building, to both your left and right are identical lifts and stairwells taking you up to the other floors. We were heading to the chemotherapy facility on the third floor – a large, open-plan room with people sitting around in comfy chairs, reading magazines, chatting to each other over coffee. The overall effect is of a large, friendly café – the only way you realise its true purpose is that every other person has a drip in their arm, attached to a mechanical pump emitting an annoying chirp every 10 minutes or so. As a result of the twin entrance arrangements, one at each end of the room, it is entirely possible to enter the room from the 'wrong' end – the one opposite to the floor's main reception. We plonked ourselves in a couple of comfy chairs and flagged down a passing nurse to say that we were here for chemo, and gave him Zarah's name. Then we sat back and waited for her name to be called.

And waited.

Over the next few hours, as we continued to wait, Zarah's grogginess intensified. Her forehead felt a bit warm. She was clammy. I mentioned this to a nurse. It's OK, someone will be with you shortly.

By 4 p.m., I was getting a bit antsy; Zarah was now asleep in her chair. Eventually, I went to find someone who looked like they might be able to help, and was astonished to find that no one 'officially' knew we were there – we hadn't been properly checked in. That was when we first learned of the existence – right down the other end of the cavernous room – of the reception desk, where you were supposed to register your arrival, at which point the chemo gets ordered, and everything grinds into action. I was told it might not actually be possible for Zarah to have chemo today as it was now so late. My heart sank. Zarah snoozed on, oblivious, as I kicked up a bit of a fuss. Eventually, a nurse came over to see her. She took her temperature. It was ridiculously high: she had another infection. No chemo today. She'd have to go to A&E for urgent antibiotics, then wait for a bed back up in the main tower. Again. Fuck. As Zarah was wheeled off through an underground tunnel to the main hospital, I called a cab to take me back to the flat to pack her an overnight bag. We were both pretty crestfallen.

For that episode, Zarah spent five nights in UCL, while they waited for the infection to clear. She was fine by Saturday, but the quickest way to get her second dose of chemo was to keep her in till Monday and give it to her on the ward.

Of course, this delay meant our trip to Slovenia would have to be postponed. Like I said, you do not get to make plans when you have cancer.

'Hi, I'd like to postpone our flights please, my girlfriend is too ill to travel at the moment.'

'No problem, sir, what sort of illness is it?'

'It's cancer.'

'Oh right. So is it "serious", or "terminal"?'

'I'm sorry?'

'If it's only a serious illness, we can only offer a partial refund. But if it's terminal, we can issue a voucher for the whole fee. So, is she terminal?'

Argh.

———

It was around this time – shortly after Zarah had been diagnosed, during the first few cycles of chemo – that we first met two wonderful junior doctors, Pramit Khetrapal and Sophia Wong, who, thanks to their interest in bladder cancer research, would go on to become fellow travellers on Zarah's journey. Both originally hail from the high-tech, multicultural city-state of Singapore, but they'd first met while studying medicine in London, and had since become good friends. Pramit, then a trainee urology surgeon, is from the country's ethnically Indian minority; Sophia, who was training to be an oncologist, is from the larger part of the population who'd initially settled from China. Neither of them was directly involved in Zarah's care (a fact that, perhaps, removed some of the usual barriers preventing patients and clinicians becoming friends). Instead, they were both, as part of their training, doing research projects based at UCL, working closely with Charlie, Mark and the others. And Zarah became their chosen subject.

It had been Sophia, earlier that month, who had collected the blood-soaked chunks of Zarah's tumour immediately after her operation at Westmoreland, and ensured their safe passage to Charlie Swanton's laboratory for analysis. And now the pair of them would regularly meet us at Zarah's monthly appointments, to collect fresh blood and urine samples for their research.

The four of us instantly struck up an easy rapport – we'd look forward to catching up with them, getting the gossip about how things were in the NHS (then in the throes of a junior doctors' strike), Pramit and

I stealing away for nerdy chats about experimental robotic surgery or obscure whiskies, Sophia regaling me with tales from the cutting edge of immunology research, Zarah and Sophia developed a particularly close bond, and the two of them would coordinate things via text message, Zarah keeping Sophia abreast of her appointment schedules to help make sure the pair of them could get a continual supply of Zarah's bodily fluids. They always seemed to be on hand when we wanted a bit of advice and support – never quite a formal second opinion, but just a friendly, clinically trained sounding board for whatever questions or issues arose – and this became invaluable over the subsequent months.

We even came up with a theme tune for them, adapted from the Paul Young classic:

'Every Time You Go Away… You Take a Bit of Wee With You.'

I want to press pause at this point, and talk a bit about chemotherapy – where it comes from, how it works (and why it sometimes doesn't), and how it's used to treat cancer. I'll try to keep it brief – after all, the subject is covered in forensic historical and scientific detail in a multitude of books about cancer (perhaps the best of which, in recent years, has been *The Emperor of All Maladies*[1] – which you should definitely read if you want to know more). But here's the potted version – a bluffer's guide, if you will.

Like many things in medicine, the discovery that ushered in the era of chemotherapy came about thanks to two things: luck and war.

The story begins shortly after the First World War – a time when cancer treatment was limited to fairly crude surgery – when a group of US researchers were searching for possible antidotes to perhaps the Great War's most infamous development: chemical weapons. As they combed through medical records from soldiers who'd been exposed to a quite horrific, blister-inducing chemical warfare agent called nitrogen mustard, they spotted something unexpected. To a man, the soldiers all had extremely low levels of immune cells in their blood, as if the chemical were specifically targeting these cells, or the body's ability to produce them. In an historic bit of outside-the-box thinking, this led them to speculate that nitrogen mustard might be effective against cancers of the immune system: leukaemias and lymphomas.

So, changing tack from chemical warfare research to cancer, they set out to test this idea. And by 1942, with another world war now in full swing, the team had gleaned sufficient evidence from laboratory studies to run human trials. At 10 a.m. on 27 August, they injected a series of doses of nitrogen mustard into the bloodstream of a patient with a large lymphoma on his jaw. Over the next few weeks, with each dose, the tumour shrank, the man's pain subsided, and he gradually regained the ability to swallow, and thus eat.

Six months later, he died, his disease too advanced, too aggressive, for the drug to contain. But despite this, his story marks the first time chemotherapy had been used to help a patient with cancer.

It was a breakthrough that would open up an entirely new field of cancer research – one that would occupy researchers for the best part of half a century: the search for chemicals even more effective against cancer than nitrogen mustard. And indeed, the world's researchers went on to uncover hundreds of such chemicals, all of which – it turns out – work by targeting a fundamental process: cell division itself.

The idea that chemotherapy targets dividing cells is, of course, extremely well known, and is part of most oncologists' explanation of why it causes its infamous side effects: diarrhoea, from its effect on the rapidly dividing cells that line your gut; hair loss, through killing your hair follicles; anaemia and infections, from its effect on the bone marrow; and so on.

What's less well known is that chemo drugs can be broadly grouped into five different classes, depending on precisely how they work. I'm going to dwell briefly on these here, partly because it's just really interesting; partly because, having spent so long talking about the science of targeted drugs in the last chapter, I don't want readers thinking that chemo drugs are any less scientifically well understood; and also, in part, because understanding how chemo works is important context to understand what makes cancer cancer.

The first broad class of chemotherapy drugs – often called DNA cross-linking agents, or alkylating agents – work directly on DNA itself, by chemically attaching small clusters of atoms to the guanine ('G') molecules in the double helix. When the cell next tries to replicate, this modified DNA plays merry havoc with the relevant machinery, breaking or jamming it. Sensing this catastrophic damage, the cell flips its suicide switch and dies through apoptosis.

This class of drug includes derivatives of the nitrogen mustard we discussed above, and – importantly for Zarah's story – a group of chemicals that all contain an atom of the metal platinum. OK, indulge me: there's a particularly cool story behind the discovery of platinum's anti-cancer properties – one that shows just how randomly lucky medical researchers can be.

In 1965, a researcher called Barnett Rosenberg was trying to find out whether electric fields could affect how bacteria grew (with one eye, one must assume, on developing new ways to treat infections). In one series of experiments, he'd happily noticed that a particular set-up caused the bacteria to stop dividing and, instead, grow into long filaments – about 300 times longer than a normal cell. Initially believing that he'd stumbled on a magical new way to fight infections with electricity, he was alas unable to repeat the finding using other equipment. It took him a while to unravel what was really going on: the electrodes he'd used were made of platinum, which was being corroded by the solution the bacteria were growing in, releasing a soluble platinum-containing chemical into the medium – and it was that, rather than the electric field itself, that was blocking the bacteria from dividing. A large quantity of laboratory mice later, he'd isolated the chemical and proved that it halted the growth of tumours as well as bacteria. Patient trials followed, and the chemical, now known as cisplatin, came into mainstream use in 1978 – the same year as Zarah was born. It's the little coincidences that really get you.

The next class of chemo drugs are called antimetabolites, and were discovered soon after nitrogen mustard. They all work by mimicking the appearance of the nucleotides that make up DNA, tricking the cell into including them as they replicate their chromosomes. Just as with the alkylating agents, these intruders cause havoc with the cell's inner machinery, and subsequently trigger death by apoptosis. The chemo combination Zarah received for her cancer included one of these drugs – gemcitabine – which masquerades as the 'C' nucleotide, cytosine.

Topoisomerase inhibitors form the third category of chemo drug, and they work by interfering with a crucial part of the cell's replication machinery – a molecular DNA detangler called topoisomerase. Blocking the action of this essential protein causes a cell's DNA to become extremely, irreparably tangled, like a Christmas Slinky in March. Apoptosis ensues.

Next up, we have the anthracyclines, and again they have an interesting origin story: they were first discovered in species of soil bacteria called *Streptomyces*, which evolved to produce them as a defence mechanism. In essence, they're antibiotics, albeit not ones you'd ever take for a cough – their side effects are absolutely horrendous. They seem to work on multiple systems within a cell – they mainly affect topoisomerase, but can also jam between rungs of the DNA helix and cause mischief, then can even cause a cell to generate DNA-damaging free radicals – highly reactive molecules that can cause untold damage if released in the wrong place. Or the right place, if you have cancer.

Finally, we have the plant alkaloids. These are – as the name suggests – a variety of chemicals isolated from plants that, again, produce them as defence mechanisms against a variety of nasties – bacteria, fungus, insects and the like. In general, they nix dividing cells by disrupting the molecular skeleton they construct during division. This stops the chromosomes lining up correctly, causing the cell to – you guessed it – flip its apoptosis switch.

By the early 1970s, cancer researchers had worked out that while a few types of cancer responded very well to chemo drugs used on their own, most only responded weakly, with resistance kicking in rapidly.

Resistance to chemotherapy is, in a dark, awful, morbid way, perhaps cancer's most fascinating and awesome superpower. It's something we so easily accept as fact that we almost forget quite how extraordinary it is. An advanced, chaotic tumour can – and almost invariably does – develop resistance to almost every form of poison oncologists can throw at it. No bacterial infection can do this, nor can viruses. Sure, resistance can develop in a population of bacteria over decades – it's why the world is about to face a crisis in antibiotic resistance – but bacterial communities pass on their resistance genes to one another by physically passing on chunks of DNA to their neighbours. Cancers work resistance out all on their own, from scratch. It's an incredible feat of biology, and understanding it is something that's occupied researchers for decades.

It turns out that cancer cells employ all manner of ingenious tricks to cope with the damage wrought on them by chemo drugs. Sometimes, they switch on molecular pumps – such as those used by liver cells to pump out toxins – and simply purge their interior of the drugs. On other occasions, they deactivate fail-safe mechanisms, allowing them to keep replicating despite the catastrophic damage to their DNA. Others switch their DNA repair mechanisms into hyperdrive, trading off the increased chances of a mistake for the ability to keep on keeping on. Others still work out how to safely metabolise the drug to a harmless form.

So, faced with the fact that single-agent chemotherapy almost always led to resistance, researchers started testing them in combinations, mixing the different classes to try to maximise the benefit. This, of course, makes sense. If you can knock out multiple different systems in a dividing cell, the chance of it developing resistance becomes lower. Unfortunately, as you increase their effectiveness, you also rapidly ramp up the side effects – and from the 1970s to the mid-1990s, spurred on in particular by dramatic successes of this approach in treating leukaemia, a vast amount of intellectual and actual manpower was geared towards finding hypothetically perfect combos of chemo – a Goldilocks-like recipe that's just toxic enough to kill all the cancer cells and avoid resistance, but not toxic enough to kill the patient.

It's unfair to say this quest was unsuccessful. Sure, many millions of people with cancer have benefited from combination chemotherapy, and cancer survival has inched ever upwards over the decades, in part due to ever more effective combinations. But the fact remains that, no matter how ingenious the combination, nor how sophisticated the dosing schedule, chemotherapy has, for the most part, proven spectacularly ineffective at eradicating cancer once it's spread. It's not, for most people with advanced cancer, a cure.* Resistance is sadly inevitable.

That's not to say chemotherapy hasn't helped cure people with cancer. It's often used in combination with surgery or radiotherapy as a sort of 'mopping up' tool, and if you look at the statistics, it's clear that, in this scenario, chemo has saved countless thousands of lives. When a surgeon removes an early-stage breast tumour, the patient has a 90 per

---

*It can, however, cure testicular cancer and some lymphomas.

cent chance of long-term survival. When the surgeon gives them chemo afterwards, that figure nudges up to around 95 per cent. Flipping that to absolute numbers, using chemo saves about five extra lives for every 100 people treated for early-stage breast cancer. The principle holds true (with different numbers) in many different cancer types. Of course, an individual patient will never know if they themselves were 'cured' by the chemo – for most of them, it won't have made a difference. And of course, all of them will have had side effects from the chemo. But such is medicine. The numbers rarely lie.

When a cancer has spread, however – when it's shot its bolt and rampaged off around the body, to the lymph nodes, to the lungs, to the liver... well, in those circumstances, all chemo can do is hold the disease at bay, kill the sensitive cells, and hope it slows the rest down long enough to do whatever it is you want to do with whatever time you have left.

With the first cycle of gem-cis chemotherapy administered (albeit somewhat chaotically and, with Zarah spending a total of eight days in a UCL bed, certainly not the relatively easy outpatient experience we'd naively expected), we tentatively looked forward to the week off before the next cycle commenced. We'd been warned that this might be a hairy few days – the chemo would temporarily cause her immune system to crash, she'd probably feel pretty zapped, but this would recover rapidly, and she'd likely be feeling much better towards the end of the cycle. So we made plans for a couple of lazy weekends, and Zarah – who didn't yet seem to be adversely affected by the chemo ('It's my Irish liver, I've been training it for this') went in to work for a few hours each day ('I don't really get much done, everyone just wants to chat to me!'); similarly, I returned to what I'd hoped would be a regular work pattern too.

Going back to the office was weird. Cancer Research UK had recently launched a new marketing campaign, aimed at both demonstrating the universality and ubiquity of 'the cancer experience' and showing how much work was going on around the UK to make things better for people with the disease. A noble sentiment; unfortunately, its physical manifestation was the plastering of the slogan 'Cancer Is Happening

RIGHT NOW' all over the country, the media and, of course, our offices. I learned to avoid the staff canteen, the walk to which was now a brutal, painful, shouty reminder of Zarah's predicament. But as a counterpoint to this, I was bowled over by the tact, sensitivity and love shown towards me by my colleagues. One thing that had kept me at the charity for so long had been the people who worked there, who I'd come to think of as a sort of extended friendship group – occasionally even as family. Now, this feeling was amplified a thousandfold. The CEO sent me a lovely text message and stopped me in the corridor to wish us well, as did several other senior staff. I was told not to worry about filling in forms for leave or sickness pay – that could be sorted later. Another colleague who had had breast cancer herself forwarded me a list of 'survival tips' for chemo to share with Zarah. I'd occasionally be stopped in the corridor for the administration of a warm, silent hug. Again, it was the kindness that would really get me, occasionally necessitating a trip to the toilets for a silent sob. The work itself was fine – almost none of it had anything specifically to do with bladder cancer, so 'trigger moments' were mercifully rare. (The only exception I can remember was when I had to sign off a comment to be issued to a journalist that opened with the words: 'The key signs and symptoms of bladder cancer are blood in the urine, but thankfully the disease can usually be successfully treated if caught early.' Bam. I calmly closed the email and forwarded it to a colleague to handle.)

The main thing occupying our team, however, was Charlie Swanton's new research paper, which was to be published slap bang in the middle of mine and Zarah's 'down week'. Charlie's team had made a phenomenally complex yet very exciting discovery. Working with some colleagues in a cancer immunology lab at UCLH, they had uncovered strong hints about the identity of the molecules on the surface of cancer cells that the immune system can 'see' (or, more accurately, feel). Moreover, if their discovery panned out, the identity of these molecules, called 'neoantigens' and which differed from patient to patient, could potentially be predicted from their tumour's warped DNA sequence, created artificially in the lab, and used to jump-start the patient's immune response against their disease. It was all highly speculative – the kind of complex science that could easily mutate into an overhyped 'cure for cancer' story if not handled with extreme care. Consequently, we'd been working on getting it right for a while – I mentioned earlier we'd commissioned a CGI graphics package, and we also had a host of other materials available to make sure journalists got the story right. I was working flat out, and having occasional surreal, rushed conversations on the phone with Charlie, which would start off discussing the animation and end up with him giving me an update on how his analysis of Zarah's own cancer DNA was going. Work/life balance, eh?

Anyway, Zarah was so far doing remarkably well – maybe it was the steroids, maybe she was just one of those people who tolerates chemo with minimal discomfort. She had a few minor mouth ulcers, was a little more tired than usual, but the expected maelstrom of nausea and vomiting failed to materialise. She even adapted quickly to life with a nephrostomy (or 'the pissbag', as we'd come to call it). The main issue she faced was her wardrobe – her skirts were generally calf-length, and her jeans were on the skinny side – neither was suitable for concealing a half-litre of fresh warm urine in a plastic bag strapped to her leg. Thankfully, we managed to adapt the netted bag-holder for her thigh, and thus bring most of her wardrobe back into use. However, we still had to have a quick 'is my nozzle showing?' check before we left the house.

So for a good – ooh – three or four days after coming home from UCLH full of that first round of chemo, things were sort of stable. Then, on the Monday of our 'week off', Zarah woke up with a sharp pain in her lower right calf.

At first, she tried to walk it off, thinking it was just a random bit of pain induced by the chemo. But by mid-morning, it had worsened, and started to get a bit hot, and red, and painful to touch. Once again, we called the UCLH hotline. Once again, we were told to head to A&E – the most likely explanation was a blood clot, caused by the chemotherapy's effect on her blood cells. This could be potentially dangerous – if the clot were to become dislodged, it could end up floating off and lodging in her brain or lungs. She'd need an ultrasound scan of her leg to investigate.

This time, being pragmatic, rather than UCLH, we decided to go to the Royal London Hospital, a mere five-minute cab ride from our flat. It was a calculated trade-off – 'The London', as it's known, has the busiest A&E department in the country, but for a quick routine ultrasound we figured it shouldn't be too much of an ordeal. We both phoned our respective employers to say we wouldn't be in today, and headed off to hospital again.

Oh, fate, why did we tempt thee so? The A&E department at The London was RAMMED. They couldn't find a slot for an ultrasound there and then, but did give Zarah a blood test, the results of which were in keeping with 'something funny going on'. They booked her in for an ultrasound, and casually told her it was almost certainly a type of clot called a deep vein thrombosis (DVT), the treatment for which, we found out, to Zarah's utter dismay, was injections with an anticoagulant drug called heparin EVERY DAY for SIX MONTHS.

So, here's a thing I haven't mentioned yet. Like Achilles and his heel, Zarah – stoic, brave, adaptable; diagnosed with cancer yet marching onwards, soaking up the sadness, smiling through everything – had a weak spot. A really, really bad weak spot, in the circumstances: she was an acute trypanophobe. In other words, she was needle-phobic: injections and needles scared seven kinds of living shit out of her.

I'd first twigged that she wasn't quite right with needles several years ago, when we were getting vaccinations before going travelling. She'd been notably quiet before heading off to the GP, and then come back white as a sheet and shaking. I'd laughed – she'd punched me in the arm. Still, I hadn't seen her phobia up close and personal until a few weeks previously, in A&E, when they had to put a cannula in her arm to get the antibiotics in via a drip. She completely Freaked. Out. Proper shaking, clenching, crying, spasming fear. 'You have cancer' – fine. 'You'll have to have an injection' – not fine at all. Of course, having cancer means lots of injections – she was dealing with this as best she could, and the nurses had all been hugely understanding and sympathetic to it – but things hadn't been easy so far.

So this new revelation – that a confirmed blood clot would mean she'd have to have **daily** injections; that of all the side effects she could have had from the chemo, she'd had a DVT – was the cruellest of all ironies. 'Henry, it's worse than having fucking cancer!' she'd told me, only in mild jest.

And of course, even confirming the DVT wasn't plain sailing. We headed back to The London the following day for an ultrasound to her lower calf... which revealed... nothing. No DVT. So did this mean no injections? Maybe, we were told. The pain was still there – Zarah was now using a crutch to get around. So the Royal London booked her in for another scan in a week's time, muttering something about the fact that they might need to wait for any clot to get bigger before it could be seen.

Later that same week, however, Zarah had an appointment for a precautionary bone scan at UCL – she popped in on the way to work (we'd quickly become so acclimatised to the seriousness of the situation that a scan to check whether her cancer had spread to her bones was something for which one could merely 'pop in'), only for the team there to look at her calf with some consternation and send her for an urgent ultrasound scan... which found a *massive* blood clot nestled behind her knee. The Royal London staff had completely missed it. She called me at my desk, in tears. She'd have to have daily injections after all. I was furious with myself not to have been with her when she got the news.

That night, I learned how to inject a grown, terrified woman in the belly with a syringe full of heparin. And over the next few weeks, we established a little routine to try to make the process as unstressful as possible. Sitting on the sofa, Zarah would lift up her top to expose her belly, turn to one side away from me, and begin colouring in one of the pages from a Jeremy Corbyn colouring book that a friend had given us as, I think, an ironic joke. I'd crouch on the floor and get into position with the syringe. Eventually, after several minutes colouring, she'd nod; I'd stick the needle in and gradually, gently, press the plunger. We'd do this every night, together, the two of us, for the next six months. It became a little ritual. I've still got the colouring book. She didn't manage to colour things in very well, but who could blame her?

While we're on the subject of injections and needle-phobia, there was one positive development on the horizon. Zarah had been reading a blog by a patient who had been undergoing a gruelling and intensive chemotherapy schedule, and who'd sung the praises of something called a 'peripherally inserted central cannula', or PICC. This is essentially a permanent cannula, fitted through a minor operation, which allows you to avoid the repeated pain and hassle of having to be cannulated each and every time you have intravenous drugs. PICCs have downsides – you have to keep them covered up in the shower, and they can get blocked or infected – but it sounded like something worth exploring.

After raising the matter with Zarah's oncology team, it was agreed that this was a sensible option for her, and an appointment was made for the operation. I was tied up at work, so she went along with her best friend, Lindsey.

Lindsey and Zarah had a very tight, almost sisterly friendship – they'd first met while working together more than a decade previously, and quickly become partners in crime, often out late together, getting involved in all manner of scrapes and shenanigans. Lindsey is enormous fun to be around – possessed not only of a razor-sharp mind and a low tolerance for fools, but also one of the dirtiest cackles known to humanity and an extremely silly sense of humour.

So it was only natural that the pair, at UCLH to have Zarah's PICC fitted, got into another of their scrapes – being busted for getting high together on the preoperative laughing gas while the doctor was out of the room, a story they recounted to me later that evening amid much cackling and mirth.

———

That week, Charlie Swanton's paper was published, and made headlines across the world.[2] At the press conference that morning, I'd chatted briefly with Charlie and his immunologist colleague Dr Sergio Quezada, a lovely, cheerful, outgoing man who I'd met a few times previously, and was helping Charlie analyse Zarah's tumour sample – 'Don't worry,' he'd said. 'We're on this. We'll do everything we can.' I'd also bumped into the charity's then chief clinician, Professor Peter Johnson, who'd been kept up to speed with events since I'd initially asked for his help some weeks previously, when they'd first discovered 'something' in her bladder. 'How are you bearing up? It's rather different on the other side of the line, isn't it?' he'd wryly observed, putting a hand on my shoulder.

Zarah's mother was staying with us at the time. The story was the lead item on the six o'clock news. While I celebrated in the pub with the team, they watched together at home – 'Look, there's Henry's team's animation.' It was odd, knowing that the man being interviewed on the telly, with my girlfriend and her mother watching, was also the man scrutinising the scrambled, chaotic sample from her tumour for ways to help her.

———

It was around this time that – over a series of phone calls, initially, surreally, bookended by discussion of his upcoming paper – Charlie had also relayed to me what he and Sergio's laboratories were learning about Zarah's cancer. Looking back, I didn't ask too many questions – I mainly wanted to know if the results gave any clues as to what might happen to her, especially whether the DNA analysis pointed towards any experimental treatment options. My broader scientific curiosity was, for now at least, relatively un-piqued.

The bad news first, delivered on my phone as I stood in one of the meeting rooms at work, speaking in hushed, nervous whispers: Zarah's tumour was not a 'good' cancer. Its chromosomes appeared extremely unstable – something often found with aggressive tumours that quickly develop resistance to treatment. And compared to the 'average' bladder tumour, the DNA had relatively few single-letter mutations – about 200-odd (compared with many thousands) – implying that it would be hard for the immune system to detect it. This latter point perhaps wasn't surprising – bladder cancers are normally found in older smokers, and have characteristic telltale signatures of tobacco-ravaged DNA, full of thousands of molecular typos. At the relatively young age of 37, Zarah was – at worst – a 'social smoker', partaking of the odd late-night cigarette but never developing a long-term habit. Whatever had led to the disease's emergence, it was unlikely to be due to years of exposure to carcinogens.

On top of this, an initial look at the number of, and nature of, the immune cells inside Zarah's tumour suggested that things were relatively quiet. It certainly wasn't what researchers describe as an immunologically 'hot' tumour – packed full of aggressive, angry immune cells called T-cells. They were planning more work to clarify what was going on here, but again, it wasn't a promising sign.

But there were also a couple of straws to clutch at. There was something going on with the tumour's *HER2* gene – the one I mentioned in the previous chapter, which makes the HER2 receptor protein. Charlie's team had spotted that the region of chromosome 17 containing this gene had been duplicated a few times, and as far as they could tell, this was an early event in the tumour's evolution. This suggested that HER2 *might* be one of the cancer's underlying drivers. This information came with an important caveat. Trials had previously looked at targeting HER2 in patients with similar bladder cancers, and these trials had been overwhelmingly negative.[3] As a result – and quite sensibly – none of the current HER2-targeting drugs routinely used to treat other cancers, such as Herceptin, could be prescribed for people with bladder cancer. Nevertheless, in Zarah's case, should other options not pan out, down the line, at some point, maybe… there might be a rationale for applying to somehow access these drugs.

The second straw was even more of a grasp, even more outlandish, but – perhaps as a result – even more of a cause for hope. Although Zarah's tumour only carried a handful of mutations, most of them were present in all the regions of the tumour. In other words, genetically speaking, the cells of her tumour were relatively uniform – often a good sign. On top of this, Charlie and Sergio's software – the very same technique underpinning their recent world-famous research – had suggested that a small number of these mutations might – *might* – mean the cells were producing neoantigens – signals that allowed the immune system to recognise them. 'We could, if you're happy with the idea, try and look and see if we can find anything,' Charlie offered.

This blew my mind. Charlie was, tentatively, with huge caveats, offering his and Sergio's help to comb through the various samples Zarah had supplied – the blood, the tumour, the urine – to see if they might be able to look for rare immune cells that had already learned how to recognise the tumour, but which – for whatever reason – hadn't been able to check its growth. And perhaps, maybe, possibly, if these cells could be found, and encouraged to grow in a lab, they could be turned into a living drug that might have the potential to attack her cancer.

Charlie was careful to emphasise what I'd already realised: the multiple pitfalls, the one-in-a-million chances, the likelihood of failure, the ethics, the bureaucracy, the unprecedented and experimental nature of the concept, and even the chances of harm. I said I'd chat to Zarah and get back to him, but I already knew what the answer would be.

And so, a plan began to emerge. The main thing: there was nothing in any of this data so far that suggested deviating from the standard evidence-based treatment protocol – chemotherapy to control the tumour as long as possible. But when that stopped working – which it inevitably would – we had a variety of options to explore. The most promising one was to try and get on a clinical trial of the immunotherapy drugs that kept making the headlines. But then also, perhaps, we might try an anti-HER2 drug, and maybe, possibly, perhaps, somehow, Charlie and co might be able to rustle up an experimental, unproven treatment based on Zarah's own immune cells.

Options. It's all you really want, with cancer. Options not to die. We appeared to have several. And for that, we were so incredibly, tearfully, gobsmackingly grateful.

Because options mean one thing above all: hope.

Things calmed down, for a while at least, for Cycle 2, and we were able to pause, catch our breath, and take stock.

We were both, naturally, pretty shell-shocked. Just eight weeks ago, at the end of a cold, rainy January, Zarah had a kidney infection – now, mid-March, as spring arrived, she had advanced cancer. She was 'a cancer patient'. And although we rarely put it in such harsh words, we both knew that the disease would eventually kill her – the big, black, Schrödinger-like box of our future contained the answer to a question that was completely unknowable: how long would we have? However long it would be, we knew it almost certainly ended with a death certificate that had the word 'cancer' on it somewhere. It was a reality and a fate we both absorbed amazingly quickly – life's dealt us a shitty hand, let's try to play it as best we can.

We also deliberately eschewed any talk of unfairness, any 'why-me?' or 'why-her?'. One evening, while watching news of the unfolding refugee crisis in Calais, Zarah remarked, 'Just think, there might be someone in those camps with a pain in their back and blood in their wee – they're not going to have UCLH, Ursula, Charlie, all that. We're the lucky ones, when you think about it.' That was quintessentially Zarah – more concerned about others than herself, always determined to see the positives.

You might have noticed that I'm talking about 'we' a lot. That's entirely deliberate – we almost exclusively talked in terms of 'we'; Zarah was adamant that this wasn't something that was happening to her, but to us. 'We' went for chemo, 'we' wondered about 'our' future, 'we' put up with the side effects. Team Twat, to the end.

Such was our shared psychological make-up that we didn't dwell too long on trying to think about time frames – at least, not with each other, or our friends. But I'm sorry to say that I kept a horrid little secret. Thanks to that fervent late-night googling back in Cork while Zarah slept, I had accidentally uncovered an inkling of what lay ahead – and it hovered at the back of my mind. While searching for something else entirely, I'd stumbled across a paper that, as an aside, mentioned the average survival time for people with stage 4 bladder cancer.

I'm not going to tell you what that number is. Not yet. We'll get to it later. I certainly didn't tell Zarah – I didn't even really dwell on it myself – it was an average, based on a large number of patients who were much older, and thus generally sicker, than Zarah was. She was exceptional, in every way – there was no way I would let that average guide my thoughts, feelings and actions. No way at all. And yet, I carried it with me throughout the whole thing. In the background. A nagging, flashing, depressing, average little light on the chaotic cancer dashboard, upon which so much else was competing for my attention.

Cycle 2 came and went as planned. We now had the beginnings of a routine – Zarah would go to work on Monday and Tuesday, have chemo on Wednesday, and take Thursday and Friday off. I'd have the Wednesdays off to go to chemo with her, but otherwise was back to work full-time. We'd go out and see friends in the evenings, have a few drinks – life was approaching 'normal', albeit a sort of limbo-like normal where making any plans further away than a few weeks was off limits. An email came round for a friend's 40th birthday in Spain in October – I'd wanted to hold off booking flights, but Zarah thought it was best to book now, when they were cheap, and cancel later if necessary.

On the weekend after Cycle 2's second dose, as its nadir approached, Zarah's older sister, Amber, came to stay, with her six-year-old daughter, Muireann. This was a long-promised trip to London for her – a Christmas present – and she was excited to see her beloved Auntie Zarah. Amber had told Muireann that Zarah was a bit ill at the moment so might be a bit tired, but 'the C word' wasn't mentioned. By this point, the chemo was indeed making Zarah pretty tired, but nothing disastrous, even given the current point in the three-weekly cycle. She had a few mouth ulcers, a few aches and pains, and wasn't sleeping that well because of the steroids. The nephrostomy bag was an occasionally embarrassing irritation, but no more than that. It would all be fine, Zarah assured me. Still, I was nervous of the arrival of a hyperactive, tantrum-prone six-year-old into our cosy cancer-bunker of a two-bed flat. I kept my anxiety to myself. In the end, it was, indeed, basically fine; we had a slightly narky Saturday where we tried to cram too much in – a local market, the Science Museum, the Natural History Museum AND the London Eye – and both Zarah and Muireann conked out in the cab home, but, looking back, it would have been terrible to have cancelled. I'm sure when she's older, Muireann will treasure those memories: she only visited her aunt once more, much later on, when things were much worse.

The following weekend, thanks to the generosity of our friends in the form of a borrowed car and the keys to an empty holiday home, we managed to escape to France – to the charming, quiet port town of Honfleur on the north coast, all winding roads and ramshackle buildings. We filled the fridge with cheese and wine, went for slow, easy walks through the ancient cobbled streets, played board games, cooked steaks. On the Saturday afternoon, my half-sister Juliane and her partner Antoine drove up from Paris, and we had lunch on the quay. Metaphorically and literally, the sun was out, and we were pottering.

But of course it couldn't last, and the clouds soon began to gather once more. Simultaneously, a dodgy *moule* gave me a violent bout of food poisoning and Zarah's groin pain – almost certainly grumbling from one of the lymph nodes affected by the cancer – started up anew, this time sharper, more acute. So our last day saw both of us miserably doubled up in pain on the sofa, scoffing painkillers, as the rain hammered down outside. My gastric woes ultimately abated, and I was OK to drive; Zarah, however, was still getting sharp stabs of pain in her lower abdomen. And this brief episode's scriptwriter had one more plot twist: I'd somehow flattened the battery on the car – by the time we'd got sorted and were on the road (thanks to some basic GCSE French – *nous sommes tombés en panne* – and a lot of gesticulating), it was a mad dash to make our appointed train. Still, though, we just about managed to cram in a high-speed, hobbling, painful tour of Calais' *hypermarché* to pick up a couple of cases of cheap French wine and a load of cheese – pain or not, nothing in the world was going to stop that from happening. We may have squabbled over which Pinot was better value. Like I said before: priorities.

Back in London, wine safely stowed in our lock-up, car dropped off, bags unpacked, calm restored, a decent night's sleep under our belt, it was time for Cycle 3, at the end of which would be a significant milestone: a CT scan to see whether the chemo was affecting Zarah's tumour.

———

As was usual before the start of each cycle, Zarah and I would see Ursula, a sort of go/no-go check-up to assess her side effects and general health, and make sure everything was going as planned. That Wednesday morning, in her small office on the second floor of the UCH Macmillan Cancer Centre, Ursula gave Zarah a gentle prod and poke… and was concerned about the sharp abdominal pain. Much more concerned, in fact, than we expected her to be. To be on the safe side, to rule out anything sinister, she wanted Zarah to have an ultrasound scan. We rolled with it, and tried not to think too hard about the implications.

Compared to other types of scan – X-rays, CT scans, MRI – ultrasound is still a pretty low-res technology. It's good for seeing the vague shapes of things, whether they're moving, whether they're liquid or solid, but that's about it. The advantage is that ultrasound uses sound waves, not radiation, so it's pretty cheap and low-risk compared to other scans. That initial ultrasound of Zarah's belly suggested three possible options causing the pain: the first was relatively benign: a hernia. The other two options were hard to distinguish on an ultrasound: a lymph node that was swollen because it was actively trying to cope with the damage being wrought by the chemotherapy; or, more worryingly, a lymph node full of new cancer cells. This meant another CT scan would be needed to investigate further. The results of Zarah's latest blood test also showed the chemo was making her quite anaemic and she'd need a blood transfusion. The upshot: just a day after our little holiday, Zarah was admitted back to the ward. Once again, I headed home to pack a bag, while she headed up to a bed on the 14th floor. More nights in hospital. More nights apart. Chemo postponed. Great. At least we'd had a holiday, I guess. The mood-o-meter swung to 'glum' – but at least the source of the pain was being investigated.

———

Thursday afternoon, however, brought fresh hell. The doctors had arrived to discuss the results of the CT scan she'd had early that morning. On the one hand, it had ruled out a hernia, and even suggested that Zarah's primary bladder tumour seemed to be shrinking – effectively a sneak preview of the mid-treatment scan. But it had opened up two contrasting possibilities about the issue in her right side.

The first option was a large blood clot – this would be a good thing, as it would imply that the chemo was wreaking havoc on the tumour in Zarah's abdomen, blowing up its cells, dissolving its blood vessels. Taken together with the apparently smaller bladder tumour, this would be really good news, especially after just two cycles of chemo.

But the other option lay down the darker end of the scale – a lymph node swelling up with rapidly growing cancer cells. This would be incredibly bad news, a so-called mixed response: although the cancer cells in her bladder were sensitive to the chemo, others in the lymph nodes weren't – and were continuing to grow. In other words, the chemo would have failed to stop the cancer progressing.

As I've said, once bladder cancer becomes resistant to chemotherapy, things get hairy pretty quickly. If this was indeed a mixed response, it was potentially disastrous news.

A few hours later, knowing they'd left us in a horrible limbo, one of Zarah's doctors swung by to try to reassure us: she'd spoken to a senior radiologist who'd had a look at the scan and felt a blood clot was more likely. Given that Zarah's entire care team were due to meet the next day to discuss all options, they wanted to do one more ultrasound scan to check – which they booked in for the following morning. We dared to hope.

The next morning, I got to the hospital early, and we waited for the porters to come and collect Zarah and wheel her down for the scan that would – hopefully – settle the matter.

———

We entered the dimly lit room together, our anxiety well suppressed behind our impenetrable positivity. The ultrasonographer was initially somewhat formal, but she soon relaxed as our daft chatter put her at ease.

Zarah lay back on the bed and lifted up her top. The woman smeared cold gel on her abdomen, and then calibrated her probe. She pressed it against Zarah's midriff; fuzzy, swirling images appeared on the screen as the probe moved, and an inaudible beam of sound waves, their passage smoothed by the gel, bounced off the tissues, organs and fluids within. And inside the machine itself, complex software transformed these echoes into images – pixelated strata of black, white and grey, crudely representing more- and less-dense regions of 'stuff' inside her.

Eventually, a dark blob appeared on screen, like a distorted Easter bunny.

'Is that her? Is that Tina?' Zarah asked.

The ultrasonographer replied, 'Oh, you've given it a name?'

'Yeah – Tina Tumour,' Zarah said with a cackle, before singing '*She's my private cancer*', while wiggling her shoulders in a terrible impression. She'd come up with the name a few weeks previously, much to the shocked hilarity of everyone she told. I'm not entirely sure what the ultrasonographer made of it, but outwardly, at least, she smiled.

Sensing our comfort and mutual ease, she began to relax and talk us through what was on the screen. 'This, coming round here past the bladder, that's the bowel.' 'So that's her poo?' 'Shut up, Henry.' 'You two! So funny.'

'So what's that?'

'That's the lymph node they want me to look at.'

Even though we knew she wasn't supposed to tell, we asked anyway.

'Well, it's hard to say. But… it looks kind of tumour-y to me.'

Whoosh. The atmosphere in the room changed abruptly. The ultrasonographer, realising she'd been caught off guard, retreated into her shell. 'Obviously, they'll need to look at this alongside the other tests,' she backtracked.

Outside in the corridor, waiting for the porters to come and wheel Zarah back up to the ward, we clung to each other and wept.

But there was a twist. With cancer, there's always a twist. That afternoon, Ursula came to see Zarah at her bedside. She saw, instantly, how distraught we were, and moved quickly to calm us down and give us the good news. The team had had a chance to look at all the pieces of the jigsaw puzzle – all of the scans together, the fact that Zarah's pain had slowly started to subside on its own – and they'd reached the opposite conclusion to the hapless ultrasonographer. Her swollen lymph nodes seemed to be filled with liquid, not cancer cells. This was a bit odd – they were pretty baffled as to what was going on, but on balance they felt that the chemo was working, and that Cycle 3 could go ahead. Ursula being Ursula, she was sure to point out that this wasn't definitive – but the best course of action was to keep pushing ahead with the chemo, and have another CT scan afterwards as planned.

Ursula also gave us some more tentatively good news: if the mid-treatment scan confirmed that the tumour was shrinking, they might be able to remove her nephrostomy and replace it with an internal stent (basically a thin plastic tube like a double-ended drinking straw) to allow her blocked right kidney to drain into her bladder as nature intended. No more pissbag. Skinny jeans ahoy.

Zarah was booked in for the first dose of Cycle 3 the following Monday, and while we waited to be discharged, we once again hugged each other and wept – this time, with tears of relief.

After the next dose of chemo, still emotionally shattered by 'it-looks-a-bit-tumour-y'-gate, we managed to escape for a bit. A friend of my mother's has a cottage in the Chilterns, a short drive outside London. She'd had breast cancer several years previously, and had spent a lot of her recovery there – would we like to use it while she was away?

It's an idyllic place – an old, converted cart shed just outside the village where the BBC's *Vicar of Dibley* was filmed. It was now early April and the surrounding woodland was carpeted with bluebells. We drove to the local farmers' market and bought a leg of lamb to roast. We did a jigsaw – a huge, glow-in-the-dark unicorn against a moonlit sky, possibly the gayest jigsaw ever – and we cuddled on the sofa in front of an open fire. The injections continued, of course. And we dared to think ahead, to maybe having a holiday later that summer, maybe, possibly, fingers crossed. Maybe.

A week later, another dose of chemo done, and I was off to New Orleans, as part of a delegation of Cancer Research UK staff attending the American Association of Cancer Research's annual conference. From a psychological point of view, I wasn't sure how wise it was to go to a cancer research conference. It was certainly a surreal thing to be doing while Zarah was right in the middle of chemo – my first break from the daily grind of hospitals, chemo and the rest; away from Zarah, but still surrounded by cancer and cancer research. But the flights had been booked much earlier, and I didn't want to cost the charity money. And perhaps subconsciously, I think I needed a change of scene. So off I went.

Charlie Swanton was there too, and we arranged to meet up. There, in a busy corridor, coffees in hand, he gave me some unwelcome news: Sergio's analysis of Zarah's tumour tissue wasn't revealing a terribly encouraging picture, and the immune system seemed to be misfiring somehow (although I wouldn't learn more about exactly how until much later).

This was important. As well as the remote possibility that Charlie and Sergio might be able to fish out some active forms of T-cell to turn into an experimental therapy – we knew that was an outside chance – our main great, shining hope was that, after the chemo was over, we'd be able to enrol Zarah on a trial of the latest phenomenon in cancer research: immunotherapy drugs called checkpoint inhibitors. These drugs work by activating the body's immune system. But for them to do so, they seemed to require the immune system to have already partially recognised the tumour's presence, and migrated to the scene of the crime; they could pull the trigger, but only if their weapons were able to fire. What Charlie and Sergio seemed to be saying was, the immune system in Zarah's tumour was heavily suppressed: as things stood, the chances of these drugs working – even if we could get hold of them – was relatively low. As, now, were my spirits.

But then later that day, by chance, I went to a talk that lifted my spirits a little. US researchers working on immunotherapy in bowel cancer had found that supposedly 'immunologically suppressed' cancers could subsequently fill up with active immune cells *after* the patient had been given chemotherapy – it seemed that as the chemo killed the cancer cells, they released signals that alert the immune system, attracting it to the tumour and laying the groundwork for the immunotherapy drugs to work later on. Given what we knew about Zarah's response to chemo – the weird swollen lymph nodes – it was just possible that this was exactly what was going on in her bladder. And a few hours later, on the way to get a sandwich for lunch, I bumped into Sergio himself. Excitedly, breathlessly, slightly tearfully, I relayed the results I'd just seen, and also what Zarah had just been through with the scans, the lymph nodes, the T-cells. He agreed – this was a promising sign: did I think there was a way to get him another sample to analyse for immune activity? I'd check, I said.

When I think back, this is such an extraordinary thing. While Zarah was at home, bravely injecting herself in the belly (she'd by now learned to do this herself – I was incredibly proud), I was on the other side of the world, surrounded by world experts in cancer, taking in the latest research, bouncing ideas off them, trying desperately to find a way through, a way to save her, to give her more time. I'd told her I'd do everything I could, leave no avenue unexplored. I was, somehow, randomly, chaotically, doing just that.

I spoke to Zarah later that night, and was careful to couch this news in the most hypothetical terms – that I'd spoken to Charlie and Sergio, that her original biopsy was a bit of a desert, immune-wise, but there was still hope, still a door we might walk through that had light on the other side. We agreed to raise the matter of a second biopsy with Ursula at the next appointment.

The conference closed a few days later, with a rousing, typically American speech from then Vice President Joe Biden. He'd lost his son to cancer, but was now spearheading a new effort to accelerate research, dubbed the 'Cancer Moonshot'. There was hope for the future. We would do this. We would defeat cancer. The delegates left the auditorium pumped and elated.

While I'd been in New Orleans finding ways to try to save her, Zarah had also had a break, heading back to Cork to see her parents, sister and a few old school friends. So we were both in good spirits by the time I got back – the break had been good, the news tentatively promising, and we were both really pleased to see each other after 10 days apart. But now it was time for the first of several big crossroads, a big reveal that would determine our futures: the results of the mid-treatment scan.

That Wednesday, as was now usual, we jumped in a cab and braved the rush-hour traffic to UCLH to see Ursula. Zarah had had the CT scan the day before, while I was still mid-Atlantic. Now we were stuck in traffic, the clock ticking. We said nothing the entire journey, inching forwards along Euston Road towards whatever fate had in store. We got there just in time, and sat nervously in the waiting area, surrounded by the hoi polloi of UCLH's urological cancer patient community. We needn't have worried – it was the middle of a junior doctors' strike, and things were running late. We glimpsed Ursula rushing between appointments – she saw us, and gave us an enigmatic smile. We did nothing but try to second-guess what it meant until Zarah's name was called.

We walked in, sat down. Ursula smiled again. 'I can see you're both nervous, so let's get it over with.'

'It looks like the chemo is working.'

Cue spontaneous, grateful tears.

Ursula brought the scans up on screen and talked us through them. There were, of course, caveats. The primary tumour, the one actually inside Zarah's bladder, was now, Ursula said, 'only about a millimetre of thickness on the bladder wall'. But this was as compared with the scan taken before Zarah had surgery, so it was impossible to tell how much of this was due to the surgeon's steel and how much from the oncologist's platinum. Either way, 'Tina' was virtually gone from the bladder for now. And, oh my word… We saw that pre-surgery scan for the very first time. Before she was diagnosed, Zarah used to joke that she had 'the bladder capacity of a walnut'. Shockingly, the scan revealed that this was literally the case – almost her entire bladder was full of cancer. No wonder the doctors in the hospital in Cork had looked at us with such pity. Zarah's tumour had been *huge*.

Next, Ursula pointed at the lymph nodes. The problematic right node, the one in the groin, had got a bit bigger, but this was the 'atypical' response we'd fretted about before – likely due to the chemo, not the cancer. But elsewhere, several other lymph nodes that had previously been swollen had now shrunk.

And finally – the lungs and liver. Still nothing. Nada.

Three cycles in, and the chemo had pruned back what the surgeon couldn't. There was still cancer there, but it wasn't going anywhere.

For now, Tina was locked in a platinum cage. The chemo – which Zarah was still tolerating with minimal side effects – would continue for another three cycles. Level One complete. Begin Level Two.

———

I want to pause again here and talk a bit about the whole idea of scans – what they are, what they mean, and why their results can be so frustratingly uncertain. After all, the idea of 'going for a scan' – for cancer, for a sore knee, whatever – is now so normal that we often don't really think about what happens when we do.

But before I get all philosophical and epistemological, some facts.

Almost all modern medical scanning involves three basic steps: first, your body, or an area of your body, is bombarded with a source of energy, which interacts with the various tissues and fluids therein. This is true whether it's a CT scan – which uses X-ray radiation; an ultrasound scan – which uses sound waves; or an MRI scan – which jiggles the body's atoms and molecules around using strong magnetic fields. Regardless of the energy source, its properties are then changed in different ways by different tissues, and these changes are collected by a detector.

Next, the detector converts this energy into electrical signals, which are fed into very clever computer programs designed to produce an image that makes sense to an actual human being.

Finally, an actual human being looks at the resulting image, and – based on what they see with their actual human eyes, and how they then interpret this thanks to their training – makes an Important Decision about what's going on in your actual human body: a decision that affects what sort of care and treatment you subsequently receive. A decision that could, literally, make the difference between life or death.

Now here's another observation. As a society, we've collectively become so accustomed to regarding digital images as True and Accurate representations of Something That Exists that we seldom pause to think about the steps that create them (steps, of course, that are very similar in standard digital photography), and how fundamentally subjective they are. Increasingly, however – perhaps because of the ubiquitous access to digital image manipulation tools – we're starting to understand how subjective this rather lazy psuedo-objectiveness can be, and realise how hard it is to make reliable decisions off the back of digital images.

But before we turn back to scans for cancer, I want to make a further point. To do so, I'm going to turn to sport, and – as I frequently do (especially when I ought to be writing a book) – to the sport of cricket.

Over the last decade or so, much debate has taken place in cricketing circles over the introduction of television replay technology to judge whether a batsman has been caught by a fielder and is thus 'out'.

In particular, in very marginal cases, using TV replays to determine whether the ball has been caught, or dropped just short, has proved incredibly hard to do – much harder, in fact, than evangelists for more technology in sport initially anticipated. This is because, far from being a True and Accurate representation of Something That Exists, it turns out that two-dimensional images can 'foreshorten' the perspective. As a result, images of balls that have just carried to the fielder look more or less identical to those that have been grassed.

Realising this problem, sports' governing bodies have come up with all sorts of rules and regulations to accommodate the fact that TV images aren't always perfect – most of which involve the input of an actual human being with experience and judgement.

And so to cancer.

Having cancer involves lots and lots of scans, images from which are used to make really important decisions. Many of these scans look for changes in things like the size, shape and density of the image of the tumour, which doctors interpret as showing whether said tumour is growing, or shrinking, or changing behaviour in some way.

Doctors, of course, know all about the inherent uncertainties in interpreting scans, so have spent literally a hundred years working out ever more reliable ways to try to do so as objectively as they can. Perhaps the most widely used criteria are known as the Response Evaluation Criteria for Solid Tumours – handily shortened to 'RECIST' (and frequently altered by my phone's autocorrect software to 'racist'). But still, ultimately – just as with TV replays and umpiring decisions – scans rely on human judgement.

And so, finally (sorry), to my point.

We as citizens – as patients, as consumers of healthcare – frequently expect a level of certainty from our doctors that is, in practice, not in their gift to give. When we get scan results (or, indeed, results from any medical test), we ultimately want to know a simple binary – is it good news, or bad? Instead, we often get shades of grey – 'It looks OK... we think'; 'It seems to have got a bit smaller'; 'On balance, we think it's probably good news'. In sport, this won't do, yet in medicine, it's the best we've got. We forget this at our collective peril.

In raising this issue, I want basically to do two things. On the one hand, I want to make a partial defence of the incredibly difficult and skilled job doctors do when they interpret a computer-generated image of the echoes of energy radiated off their patient's body's tissues, and then convey to the patient what this means for, essentially, their estimated lifespan. We often don't quite think through – at least, I didn't to start with – what a tricky tightrope this is to walk, especially when scans aren't clear-cut. No scan is ever as accurate as physically cutting a patient open and looking at their tumour – which quite obviously isn't a desirable way to do medicine.

But on the other hand, I also want to say this to the doctors out there: the language you use when talking to your patients about their scan results *really* matters – particularly given the inherent subjectivity surrounding what scans really are. The best doctors – and, for the most part, Zarah's doctors really were some of the best – get this, and try to allow for the uncertainty, framing things appropriately and sensibly. But I've heard too many stories about doctors whose patients don't quite understand what scans really show, and who, by failing to properly explain the shortcomings of modern medical imaging, have caused upset, uncertainty, and fear – and that's as much their responsibility to get right as it is their patients' to understand.

Right, that's my scan rant out of the way. Back to the story.

I can't emphasise enough how the news that the chemo appeared to be working – that Zarah's tumour was apparently stable, and wasn't spreading anywhere new – transformed our outlook. We'd been told that there was a fair chance of a response – around two-thirds of aggressive bladder cancers like Zarah's do, apparently – but in retrospect, we'd failed to properly engage, at least on a conscious level, with the idea that Zarah's might be in the *other* third. Now, even though we were only halfway through the treatment, the revelation meant we could – and did – begin to think tentatively about things like 'holidays' and 'Christmas'. Phrases like 'next year' re-entered our daily vocabulary. We were, all things considered, pretty chipper.

Of course we were still cautious. Of course we tried to keep our feet on the floor. But after the previous three months of relentless uncertainty and wildly oscillating emotions, having some tangible good news was just what we'd needed. And our newfound optimism and good cheer spread throughout our wider circle of friends.

By now it was late April, and spring was well sprung. The evenings were sunny. We'd meet friends for picnics in the park. We were doing 'normal stuff' again.

These good spirits continued as the final three cycles of chemotherapy passed, in the main, without much incident. Zarah was never one to take prescription drugs unnecessarily, so she scaled back her anti-nausea steroids to the bare minimum. And so the unpredictable mood-altering effect of the steroids was minimised. OK, she still got a bit knackered from time to time, had an occasional whiff of nausea, and, thanks to the chemo, her taste buds had 'gone weird' (she now found red wine undrinkable. Thankfully, a good G&T still hit the spot). But her pain was well controlled thanks to daily low-dose morphine tablets, and outwardly she was back to something like her normal self.

As a result, people would say things like, 'Wow, you'd never know Zarah had cancer', which would be simultaneously lovely to hear and also like a little dagger to the heart. The outward normality was still coming at a price, physically and emotionally – especially for Zarah. Living with cancer sucks. Physically, the heparin injections continued (the colouring book was now quite a state). Sleep was still disrupted. There was still a plastic nephrostomy tube running from her back to a bag of piss strapped to her leg. The continual morphine, relief though it was, brought some fairly hefty constipation in its wake. And emotionally, although things were unimaginably better than before the scan, our future was still a big black box suspended in time and space. But for now, none of this mattered, really, because we were here, and alive, and in love. In mid-May, we celebrated my 39th birthday in traditional drunken fashion. We didn't talk much about the next one – the big four-oh. Why tempt fate?

Zarah was soon able to leave behind another of these 'inconveniences'. In late May she went back into Westmoreland Hospital to have her nephrostomy 'internalised' – in other words, the external drainage bag was to be replaced by a thin internal tube inserted down her ureter, through Tina, and into her bladder. The doctors were really cautious in managing our expectations – they'd seen the scans, knew how much tumour was still there, and were keen to stress that they'd try their best, but there were no guarantees they'd be able to get the stent through successfully. But Zarah was convinced it would work, that the caveats were just 'responsible doctoring'. 'I'm telling you, Henry, this bag's going to be gone by tomorrow,' she'd said. 'They're just trying to manage my expectations, but I can tell they think it'll be OK.' I'd worried she was pinning too much on success, investing too heavily, setting herself up for a fall.

I needn't have worried. She woke up from the operation sans nephrostomy, and we cheered. She always was so great at reading people – even hard-to-scrutinise medical professionals, it seemed.

It's hard to overstate how much of a change the loss of the nephrostomy had on Zarah's quality of life. Imagine, if you will, that every time you get out of a seat, or have to hurry along a bit quicker than you need to, or want to roll over in bed, you have to pause, and check yourself, and worry that a little coiled tube is going to be yanked painfully out of your kidney. Or that the nozzle will catch and release half a litre of urine on to your clothes. Or just that people are staring at that funny loop of yellowy plastic tube protruding from the hem of your skirt. Getting rid of the nephrostomy was HUGE, and added to our growing sense that things were improving, that we were over the worst, that there were good times ahead.

It was also around this time, in one of our appointments with Ursula at UCLH, that we had our first conversation about what would happen after chemotherapy – now just weeks away.

The conventional approach was to zap the tumour with some radiotherapy to try, in Ursula's words, to 'consolidate' the effects of the chemo. But the real prize, as far as I was concerned, was to try to get Zarah on to a trial of one of the new generation of immunotherapy drugs that were generating such excitement among doctors and commentators worldwide. This had the tangible prospect of kicking things into touch for far longer than anything conventional treatments could achieve. There was real hope, and we were hoping it.

But for this to happen, it would require various stars to be in alignment: namely, that such a trial would have to be actively recruiting UK patients, and Zarah would have to fit its eligibility criteria. Neither of these things could be guaranteed. And of course, the drugs would have to work – something they didn't do in the majority of patients. Nevertheless, it was an option previous generations of bladder cancer patients just didn't have.

There was a further complication too: we'd have to switch hospitals and leave the comfortable familiarity of the staff at UCLH. According to Ursula, the main centre in London running trials of immunotherapy for bladder cancer was St Bartholomew's Hospital in Farringdon – conveniently not too far from our East London flat, and substantially nearer than UCLH. Ursula agreed to begin exploring this option, and it was during this conversation that we first heard mention of Barts' clinical trials head honcho – Professor Thomas Powles, later to become a central figure in our lives; all we knew of him at that stage was that he had a non-intuitively pronounced surname ('Poles', to rhyme with Beyoncé's surname). But let's not get too far ahead, there's LOADS to talk about before we get to the magnificently quirky genius of Tom Powles.

We'd also had some other, less conventional good news, from an unexpected quarter. Sophia – one of the researchers studying Zarah's blood and urine samples – had made a potentially exciting observation. After Zarah's second cycle of chemo, at more or less the same time that her lymph nodes started behaving painfully weirdly, her blood started to contain large numbers of highly active T-cells – the sort that are involved in tracking down and destroying cancer cells. Sophia had found that these all bore high levels of a molecule called PD-1 on their surface and, importantly, were also producing a protein called granzyme B – a membrane-puncturing protein used to destroy damaged cells, suggesting they were primed and ready to fire. She was at pains to stress that there could be a number of possible explanations, but the most obvious one was this:

As the cisplatin chemo assaulted the cancer cells in Zarah's bladder, the cells were bursting open, releasing their molecular innards into Zarah's bloodstream. This oncological debris was acting much like blood in a shark pool, waking up the immune system to the damage in the bladder and drawing it towards its origins. Given what we'd previously been told – that Zarah's tumour was immunologically suppressed – this discovery gave us tentative hope on two fronts: first, that Zarah's immune system was now becoming actively engaged in trying to contain her disease, and second, that if and when she *did* get hold of some immunotherapy, there was a greater chance of it working.

As May turned to June, the weather continued to improve, along with our spirits. We neared the final dose of the final cycle of chemo and whatever lay beyond. But cancer being cancer, there was one final twist before the chemo was done. My oldest childhood friend, Kieran – a professional musician – had given us VIP tickets to a music festival taking place in Victoria Park, just a stone's throw from our flat. We were pretty excited – the line-up looked amazing, and the two of us loved a good festival. Naturally, the morning of the event, Zarah woke up with a fever. Taking no chances, we went straight to A&E, and thence back up UCLH's tower to a bed on the 14th floor. Over the next 24 hours, poor Zarah went steadily downhill – it was a really nasty infection this time – and she spent most of the weekend dozing before the antibiotics finally kicked in.

It rained the entire weekend. Schadenfreude can be a powerful tonic, we joked on Sunday evening as our friends texted tales of muddy queues and damp squibs while we looked out across a rainy London from the 14th floor of UCLH. No wellies for us. Drips, blood tests, NHS food, and a strip-lit oncology ward... but no wellies.

There was an added twist of anxiety with this infection too, that bears dwelling on. The doctors had no doubt that Zarah had an infection – her blood markers were pretty conclusive on this. The issue was *where*, and this was a question upon whose answers rested some fairly crucial decisions.

There were three potential sources – her chemo-blasted bladder; the stent in her kidney; or her PICC line. If the infection was in the bladder, it was no real big deal – we'd just have to wait for the infection to clear. But if her stent was infected, it would mean an operation to replace it – more hospital time, more appointments. Similarly, if it was the PICC, it would also have to be replaced and – setting off Zarah's intense needle-phobia – her imminent final round of chemo would have to be given via a cannula. We hoped that the bugs were in her bladder.

To investigate, the nurses took a urine sample and drew some blood from her PICC, and sent both samples off to the labs to see if any bugs could be cultured from them. This – despite all the advances we have in technology – is still the standard way hospitals identify infections (and thus decide on the best course of antibiotics), but it has a big drawback. It can take several days for bacteria to appear in the culture. More waiting. And, of course, there are some bugs that will grow happily in a human, but much less so in a hospital lab – so a negative result doesn't *necessarily* mean no infection… In an era where we can put man on the moon, access the sum total of human knowledge from a hand-held smartphone, all the rest of it, it seems that medical science can't pin down the source of infection in the human body without taking bits of it and waiting several days for them to go off. In an era of high-tech imaging and next-generation DNA analysis, it seemed to me to be an infuriating gap in contemporary medicine.

Even more infuriatingly for Zarah, snoozing sweatily in a hospital bed, drifting in and out of consciousness, absolutely *nothing* grew from either sample. This would mean further investigation. She was sent for a scan to see if there was any telltale inflammation visible around her stent. More blood and urine was taken to have another crack at growing things in the lab. More waiting. More uncertainty. More worrying about more needles.

Then, almost overnight, thanks to the generic antibiotics they'd pumped into her body in the meantime, the infection cleared up all by itself. We never got to find out where it was, and it didn't matter any more. Zarah was back in the room, chatting away. She was given her final round of chemotherapy on the ward that Friday, after spending nearly a week in hospital. Another milestone reached. 'Last one going in now,' I excitedly emailed our friends and family as the toxic chemicals infused her body for the final cycle (such was our joy, we didn't even stop to think about the longer-term plan).

And finishing chemo meant another positive development. Since she was no longer full of blood-thickening chemo, Zarah's doctors decided to risk switching her from daily heparin injections to a brand new tablet-based anticoagulant called rivaroxaban, which had recently come on the market. It hadn't been fully tested in patients taking chemo, but given the effect of the injections on Zarah's overall quality of life, the doctors felt it was a risk worth taking. We were hugely grateful. No more daily injections. No. More. Daily. Injections.

So that Friday, after five nights in UCLH, armed with another sack of drugs from the pharmacy, including the magic anticoagulant pills, we headed home and packed to go away for the weekend to see some friends.

We left the colouring book behind.

———

The week after Zarah finished chemo was the first of a new, uncertain future. For us, it was our first without the looming prospect of more chemotherapy. For everyone else, it was the week the UK voted to leave the European Union.

Zarah and I were both passionate 'Remainers', and Zarah, being an Irish ex-pat, had particularly keenly felt the benefits of EU membership – the Celtic Tiger had roared during her youth, the Troubles had abated thanks in part to the safety net of the European Courts, and of course, being an EU national meant she could live and work in this country without hassle. But another EU reality had reared its head when we'd gone to France a few months earlier: thanks to our European Health Insurance Card, we'd not had to worry about healthcare while we were away. If anything flared up, we knew we could simply walk into the nearest hospital and be treated for free. The prospect of losing this – and thus the ability to travel hassle-free in the EU – gave our pro-Europeanness an added urgency.

The night of the referendum itself, I was abroad with work for a few days, at another research conference – this time in Portland, Oregon. It's a night I'll never forget. The obligatory end-of-conference dinner was an odd affair – all the Brits in the room ignoring the keynote speaker, gazing at their phones – the time difference meant the result was still a few hours off, but the early results were not good. We retired to the hotel afterwards, and I called Zarah in London, where she was staying up with some friends to await the result. We were still talking when it came in. Devastated, we shut up and she turned the TV up so I could hear David Dimbleby announce that the world had changed. Fuck. We lost.

2016 – what a year.

After I rang off, angry and bewildered, I headed back to the hotel bar, where a few colleagues, including our then chief executive, Harpal, were drowning their sorrows. I ended up engrossed in conversation with him – talking first about Brexit, then about Zarah. I'll always remember the kindness he showed me while I wittered on.

Despite the post-Brexit gloom (and lots of shouting at the telly), we were still in pretty good spirits over the next couple of weeks. So good, in fact, that we did something that, in retrospect, seems almost surreal. We met with an estate agent and went to look at a flat.

Zarah had long wanted a dog – and that meant moving somewhere with a garden. We'd worked out that, if I sold my flat, her salary at M&S meant we could get a joint mortgage large enough for us to afford somewhere not too far from where we lived in East London (neither of us wanted to move out of London), and she was absolutely adamant that we at least have a look at what was out there. All sorts of questions buzzed around my head – could we *really* afford it? Wasn't the economy about to crash? Can you even *get* a mortgage with stage 4 cancer? (The answers will remain forever unknown – we stayed put in the end.) But the joy of thinking about a future together, starting from scratch, having a garden, a cat… I mean, a dog (we never really agreed on that) meant I pushed it all to one side and indulged in the fantasy world of moving house. I mean, moving house while Zarah had cancer, what were we thinking? I know exactly what we were thinking, although neither of us wanted to say it out loud. The flat was beautiful. We went for a pint afterwards, and talked excitedly about the future, ignoring the massive cloud of uncertainty hanging directly above our heads.

There was a final coda to this chapter: the post-chemo CT scan, which would define just how well Zarah had responded to the chemo. In defiance of everything being written in the press about the need for a '24-hour NHS', Zarah had the scan itself on a Sunday. We were due to get the results the following Wednesday. This was an ordeal in itself, not much different from the one she'd had halfway through chemo. Once again, we got stuck in traffic and nearly had a meltdown. Once again, before the appointment we caught Ursula's eye in the waiting room and spent the whole time trying to interpret her look. And once again, we sat down nervously in the chair in Ursula's room, firmly clasping each other's hand, to find out what the future held.

The results were frustratingly inconclusive – but, thankfully, broadly positive. The good news: there was no sign of any new growth anywhere else – neither in her kidneys, liver nor lungs, nor were any new lymph nodes in her abdomen affected. And the residual primary tumour in her bladder had stayed completely stable, still visible as a slight thickening of the bladder wall. All very encouraging.

However, the two main lymph nodes on the left and right of her bladder were still swollen and, if anything, had got *very* slightly bigger. But the key thing was that they still had what Ursula described as a weird 'fluidy, cysty look' to them, rather than appearing as a solid mass – in other words, they didn't look like lymph nodes typically do when they're full of cancer cells. I'm obviously no radiologist, but Ursula showed us the scan, and you could clearly see the actual nodes themselves in solid dark grey and then, much lighter, large bulbous spherical masses ballooning out of each. This had, apparently, proven really difficult for the radiologist to interpret – it could either be some abnormal tumour growth (and hence slight progression), or conversely it could be an atypical reaction to the chemo that would resolve over time. The only way to tell for sure, Ursula said, was by sitting back and waiting, and doing another scan in a month or so's time. Such is the nature of cancer, and of scans. Nothing is certain, everything is subjective. Wait and see what happens.

Uncertainty aside, the main take-home message Ursula wanted us to absorb was this: it could be much, much worse. Tina was very much under control.

You might think that we'd leave the room flying high. But the thing I remember most, which completely dampened my enthusiasm, was something Ursula said, the implications of which I don't think Zarah really got. She told us that now was the time to think about going on a long holiday. 'You've been through the wringer. Go and have some fun,' she said.

We'd got a couple of breaks planned, Zarah told her. Next month, a trip to the countryside then a long weekend in Spain. In August, a music festival, then 10 days in France in September.

OK, said Ursula, but you could definitely do something bigger if you wanted. Zarah thought she was talking about the safety of her travelling abroad, but I got what Ursula really meant. This might be your last holiday. Make it count.

But for once, the implications, the dynamic, the mood, sailed right over Zarah's head.

In the cab on the way home, I suggested that maybe we reconsider – think about something bigger, longer, further away. It was met with fury. I think it was the only proper row we had throughout Zarah's whole illness. 'We've been fucking planning this for ages, why the fuck do you want to change things now?' She was properly angry, incomprehensive of why I was having a change of heart.

'Well, Ursula might have meant…'

'What? What do you mean? I'm not about to drop dead, you know.'

I think Ursula meant you might not have long left – I didn't say. Instead, I changed the subject.

4

Annabell's story

WE ARE INDEED GOING to change the subject – at least, sort of: I want to wind the clock back a bit, and tell you a different story now – a parallel story that intersects with our own. Because Zarah's diagnosis wasn't the first time cancer had encroached into our lives.

They say one in two people develop cancer at some point in their lives. They never tell you which one, though.

Nor when.

———

'Free Books!' If you're British, over a certain age and used to get the Sunday papers every week, you'll probably have been aware of Book Club Associates – by output, if not by name. Their schtick was simple. You'd spot one of their prominent, glossy adverts in the Sunday supplements. Eager to get a free copy of one of the latest bestsellers it offered, you'd sign up to a genre-based 'book club', who'd post it to you, in return for your signature on a contract. Under the terms of said contract, each month you'd receive a glossy magazine detailing the latest books in the genre – all at low! low! prices – from which you'd be obliged to buy a couple. Every month. Forever.

It was a genius idea, and – for a considerable time – a successful one. From small beginnings in the 1960s, the company had, by the 80s, grown to become the largest mail-order book retailer in the UK, operating more than 20 separate specialist book clubs covering everything from aviation to murder mystery.

By 2004 – six years before we met – Zarah was working as an Associate Editor at BCA, producing the regular magazines for a couple of their book clubs – one covering 'mind, body and spirit', the other focusing on science fiction.

And it was there, at their North London offices, that she had first met Annabell.

'I actually remember the day vividly,' Annabell told me. 'It was my first day there, in January, the first working day after the Christmas break. Zarah had already been there for a few years, so she took it on herself to show me around, and took me out to lunch with the rest of the team. We went to the Chinese on Camden High Street, and they brought me up to speed on the goings-on of the company, in a way that... let's say, wasn't in the formal induction handbook.' And at the end of Annabell's first day, the whole team ended up in the pub.

On any given working day at BCA, ending up in the pub was pretty much a given – and Zarah was invariably the chief instigator. 'It was a big company, with lots of young employees, so there was a lot of after-work socialising,' Annabell says. Even though there were a lot of different cliques, Zarah was somehow part of them all. She was also good friends, of course, with the landlords of the local pub – who were Irish.

Almost immediately, Annabell and Zarah became friends as well as colleagues. Zarah introduced her to her non-work crew, with whom Annabell started hanging out regularly.

'At the time I started at BCA, I'd already got a ticket to Glastonbury. Zarah was going too, and her lot had space for a lift – and I ended up camping with them, rather than the people I'd bought tickets with.' It was a bonding experience – Glastonbury with Zarah was, in general, a Herculean task of endurance and lack of sleep, from which it could take weeks to recover. It was also ridiculously good fun, and an experience that would cement their growing friendship. 'Building up to that, because I was living with my parents in the suburbs of London, I sometimes couldn't be arsed to go home after the pub, so would stay at her flat from time to time. She just kind of opened her arms to me, I guess,' Annabell says.

Also part of this warm, alcohol-fuelled, Irish embrace were a number of other BCA employees – Lindsey, Becky, Suzy and Kesh – who, along with Annabell and Zarah, formed a tight-knit group. And shortly after meeting Zarah, they became my friends too – they still are.

It was a deep, close friendship group, and would outlast all of their time at BCA: one by one, their careers moved on.

In fact, the group would even outlast BCA itself. As with many companies of that era – especially in the publishing world – it collapsed amid the white heat of the Internet revolution. After multiple buyouts and changes of owners, it finally went bust in 2012, unable to adjust to the digital era.

In April 2013, a year after BCA's collapse, things for Annabell also took a downward turn.

'I was training for a half-marathon. I was training quite a lot and I was really into it. And I noticed this... mole on the back of my calf. It was growing, I kind of knew it was growing. I didn't really want to think why. And I'd noticed that it had started bleeding if it got nicked while shaving my legs, and that was happening more and more. So I knew I needed to call a doctor, but waited until the Monday after the race. I feel like an idiot about it, but I think a lot of people do in that situation, so I have to accept that.

'And when I saw the doctor, she said right away, "I think this is something we have to worry about".'

Annabell's GP referred her to a specialist at the local Homerton Hospital. 'I think she mentioned cancer, I think she had to. I was like, OK – I guess at that point still not really wanting to accept it. And then the appointment came quite quickly, and when I saw the dermatologist she was like, "We need to get that out right away, we need to take as much out of it as we can, I'm 98 per cent certain it's melanoma".'

The Homerton is a teaching hospital, and for Annabell's appointment, the dermatologist was accompanied by a medical student, who would observe and take notes. And as the former took a scalpel to Annabell's calf, she relayed proceedings to the latter – and also, inadvertently, disconcertingly, to Annabell, who was lying down, facing the other way. 'She basically kept saying, "We need to go deeper, we need to take more out, we need to keep on going." This was right after being told that it's probably melanoma, and being given a few sheets of printed information… it was quite a lot to take in,' she says, with characteristic grace and understatedness.

The dermatologist had removed as much of the suspect tissue from the leg as possible, then bandaged up the sizeable, anaesthetised wound. And then a shaken, bewildered Annabell went home. She hadn't planned to.

'I'd cycled to the appointment, I was going to go to work afterwards – I was just like, oh, it's just a morning appointment, I'll be there two hours later. But after the operation, they told me I wasn't allowed to cycle, or run, or stretch in any way for about two weeks. So I had to walk my way back home, change my clothes – because I then had a big bandage on my leg and my jeans wouldn't fit over it – and then go back to work.

'I also called my mum then, and was honest with her about what they'd said, and then I knew that that meant the rest of the family would know pretty much straight away, because that's how our family works. We're really close. She was like, "Oh my God… do you want me to come over?" But I told her, no, I'm going to work, which she thought I was mad doing… but what else was I going to do?'

And so, three years before Zarah's journey began, Annabell's own had started.

She told Zarah about it a month later, during dinner for my birthday in a shabby, kitsch pizza restaurant on Bethnal Green Road. It was the first time we'd seen her for a while because, by coincidence, Annabell had had a terrible bout of cystitis, and the antibiotics she'd been given had caused her to react really badly.

'I'd lost tons of weight, I couldn't eat, I couldn't drink anything, I wasn't hungry, everyone was fussing about it, especially my mum. Up to that point, it was the most physically unwell that I'd ever been – a whole week of being properly sick. So actually, to me, at the time, that was more of a worry.'

After recounting the whole antibiotics saga to Zarah over a pizza, she added, almost as an afterthought, the situation with her leg. 'Zarah was just like, "What the fuck", like, "Why haven't you told me this before?" and she was very concerned straight away.

'Actually, I remember being surprised by how concerned everyone else was – everyone seemed really concerned that I wasn't worried, and I was concerned that they were worried. I remember that quite specifically.'

Later that night, after we got home, Zarah told me tearfully what Annabell had told her. I remember thinking two things: fuck: melanoma, that's not good. But also that, in its earlier stages, surgery could cure it. And, for the first of what would turn out to be many, many times, I reassured Zarah: everything would be OK.

Shortly after that, Annabell went to the melanoma clinic at the Royal London Hospital, for another, deeper operation on her leg, and to take a couple of lymph nodes from her groin, to look for any signs that the cancer had spread. She was told the results a few weeks later.

'One of those lymph nodes came back positive,' she remembers – and this necessitated another, even more extensive groin operation to remove all the nodes there. It was a frustrating time and, without a formal diagnosis of how far the disease had spread, Annabell was stuck in limbo.

'It was always, at that point, "We need to do this, we need to do this, we need to keep investigating". There wasn't like, a "This is your diagnosis", it was "We need to check something. OK, now we need to check something else".'

In early September, she thought she'd got an answer: the number of affected nodes in her groin meant her disease was stage 3B – fairly advanced, but containable. But then, a few weeks later, the doctors spotted a second suspicious mole near the top of her leg. She had it removed and a sample sent for tests. It, too, was a melanoma. And Annabell's diagnosis was upgraded to stage 3C.

'I'm not the sort of person who asks doctors too many questions – I didn't really want to know what stage it was,' she says. 'Especially since, any time I did ask, it seemed to go up. Which is kind of not really the way medicine's supposed to work – but that's cancer for you, isn't it?'

But despite the 3C diagnosis, Annabell's immediate treatment was over. She'd be closely monitored, but the melanomas had been removed, along with the affected lymph nodes. She was, as far as medical science could tell, cancer-free.

Around the same time as Annabell was processing this news, I went to a research conference, where – quite by chance – a melanoma specialist was speaking about the need for better ways to assess how far a patient's disease had spread.

'Take stage 3C melanoma,' I remember her saying. 'We call it the 50:50 disease. Half your patients, you cut out their cancer and that's it. They're cured. You never see them again.

'And the other half come back a year later, covered in aggressive melanomas. And there's really not a lot you can do.'

I remember sitting there at the time, shocked and slightly teary. Over the years I'd become used to the cold, academic tone adopted by clinical researchers at such events, but given Annabell's situation, hearing this information, and being able to interpret it so personally, was a completely new experience for me – the researcher's sober insight was the first time that abstract cancer statistics had crashed, unexpectedly, into the potential fate of someone I was close to.

It was not an insight I chose to share with Zarah. Nor with Annabell. In fact, I tried not to think too much about it myself.

Over the next few months, life for Annabell gradually returned to something close to normal, and she started to think of cancer in the past tense, as something she'd *had*. That's not to say everything was fine and dandy – the operation to remove the lymph nodes in her groin had meant she'd developed a condition called lymphoedema, causing her leg to swell up with excess fluid. (We'll come back to lymphoedema later, but – for now – all you need to know is that it's a common, uncomfortable, under-acknowledged and very difficult to manage side effect of cancer treatment – and sometimes, of cancer itself.)

'The lymphoedema was very bad at the beginning, but they couldn't formally diagnose until it had been going on for a certain amount of time,' she says. Eventually, she was referred to a lymphoedema clinic and fitted out for a specialised stocking to limit the swelling.

'And then it was very much like, OK, that's happened, now I need to get on. I went back to job hunting, I went back to trying to date, trying to deal with all the things I'd had to shelve for a while because I was thinking about cancer.'

But it was to prove a brief respite – the eye of melanoma's hurricane. Eight months later, in July 2014, Annabell noticed a few strange acne-like spots around the scar on her leg. 'I thought it was something to do with the lymphoedema, so I went to see the nurses to check, and they were like "We need to get you back to dermatology right away". They made the appointment the next week. And they took one look and said, "OK, this is a recurrence".' They took a biopsy to confirm their suspicions and sent it for tests.

The 50:50 disease.

As Annabell waited nervously for her biopsy results, her life also took a happier twist. She went on a date with the man who would, much later, become her husband – James.

The pair hit it off instantly. Another date followed swiftly, and then, just before their third date, she got the news she was dreading: the cancer had definitely come back, and she'd need further treatment – a relatively new, localised procedure called electrochemotherapy, in which a chemotherapy drug is injected into the site of recurrence, then zapped with an electric current to help the cells absorb it.

But first, she had to tell James.

'I really liked him. We were messaging each other all the time. So I thought, OK, if I want to carry on seeing him I have to tell him what's going on, otherwise I can't have this relationship with him. And also, partly I thought maybe he can come back to mine, but I've got this massive gaping hole in my leg, so I'll have to tell him. So we went out on a Friday night and I told him.'

His response: simple, understated, and very British:

'Oh blimey.'

Well, what else do you say?

'But then he asked some questions, the kind of questions that made me think, OK, he's not scared of this, he's actually just asking how I'm living with it all. Which was quite unusual, because a lot of people, when I first told them about it… friends, colleagues, family, they didn't, kind of… handle it in that way,' she says. Later that evening, he went back to hers.

It turned out that they had a lot in common – both had grown up in a similar area of London; James's sister had worked with Annabell before they'd met; Annabell's flatmate at university was a friend of James's from sixth form.

Much, much later, they would discover that their links went even deeper than they'd initially thought.

James's mother's name is Miriam – the same as Annabell's grandmother. As James told me, 'My nan named her children after people who made an impression on her, and we knew that Mum was named after a girl in her class who had red hair, who was called Miriam.

'Eventually, we put two and two together, and through talking to our relatives, worked out that the girl with red hair was Annabell's grandmother. And that my mother is named after her.'

As their relationship gently blossomed in the face of an anxious, uncertain future, Annabell turned back to face the building storm.

But despite several rounds of electrochemotherapy, the spots around the scar on her leg kept coming back. And then, the day before New Year's Eve, she noticed the scar at the top of her leg, where the second melanoma had been removed, was doing something odd too.

'I said to James, "OK, we have to go see the doctor." I got the first appointment after New Year. And they said straightaway, "We know what that is, we don't have to biopsy it."

'And that was when they first started talking about immunotherapy.'

In particular, they wanted to give Annabell a brand new drug, called ipilimumab.

In April 2014, I'd just returned to Cancer Research UK after seven months on sabbatical, travelling the world with a then very much fit and healthy Zarah. On my first day back in the office, I'd bumped into the charity's then chief clinician, Professor Peter Johnson, in a corridor. He'd greeted me warmly – we've always got on fabulously – and I asked what had been happening in my absence.

'Oh, you know, same old, same old,' I remember him saying, 'except, who'd have thought it: it looks like immunotherapy might actually work!'

Up until that point, cancer immunotherapy – treatments that harness the immune system to detect and destroy cancer cells had had a long, frustrating and yet fascinating history. And to really get your head around it all, just as before, you need to know some basic concepts about how the immune system works in general.

So, without further ado, here's Another Science Bit.

As a third-year undergraduate, I remember sitting in a university lecture theatre listening, slack-jawed, as the lecturer explained, over a series of talks, how the different parts of the immune system cooperate, and about the molecular machinery that operates inside and between our cells to help it. It was as awe-inspiring and headache-inducing then as it is now: a system that started to evolve early on in our biological history (primitive sponges contain immune-like processes to prevent them being colonised by their neighbours) and which – in complex animals like humans – has now evolved into an incredible network of hundreds of different types of cell, all of which are manufactured by your bone marrow, and nurtured and stored in organs like your spleen, lymph nodes and thymus.

Together, these tightly controlled cells carry out an extraordinary range of functions that keep you alive. Most obviously, they defend you against harmful bacteria, viruses and other nasties. But they also regulate wound healing, inflammation and blood clotting, and tend – shepherd-like – to the multitudes of essential bacteria your body contains, known as your microbiome. Clearly, all of the immune system's various abilities, including its destructive firepower, need to be switched on only in the right place, for the right amount of time, in the right way.

Let's look at some of its key players – three principal cells of the immune system – which can be grouped into two main types, then subdivided, almost fractal-like, into yet more subtypes.

First are the phagocytes, and the most important of these – for our story at least – are the macrophages: large, wobbly, highly mobile cellular garbage disposal units that wander around our tissues, eating up and breaking down a wide variety of cellular debris, including dead and dying cells and – should they encounter any – harmful bacteria and other invaders. Also important are the dendritic cells – sentinel-like entities that, like macrophages, wander the body absorbing fragments of dead cells, but, rather than digest them, instead they transport their contents back to the lymph nodes. Here, they physically present them – on their surface – to other immune cells, to see if what they've brought home is worthy of an immune response (we'll come back to this later).

The second type of immune cell – even more important for our cancer story – is the lymphocyte, of which there are two main types.

B-lymphocytes, or B-cells, secrete soluble, sticky proteins called antibodies – and each of the hundreds of thousands of different B-cells in your body is programmed to make a single type of antibody, each of which has a different target – known as an antigen. The word 'antigen' is a catch-all term, and can be almost anything – a small region of a giant protein, a fragment of DNA, a complex chain of carbohydrates – but most often, it's a short chain of amino acids called a peptide.

When an antibody sticks to its target antigen – whether it be part of a bacterium, a protein made by a virus, or part of a dying cell – it effectively labels it for destruction by other immune cells, notably the macrophages we met earlier.

Our B-cells' repertoire of antibodies is quite extraordinary, and understanding how each of us is born with a unique, sophisticated molecular recognition system – capable of responding to practically any type of invader, despite never having encountered it before – has taken many decades, and yielded several Nobel Prizes. The short story is this: your chromosomes contain several antibody genes, each of which has a highly unstable and variable region that encodes the part of the antibody protein that actually binds its target. When you're developing in the womb, an ingenious two-step process occurs in your developing bone marrow. First, in the nascent population of B-cells, these genes are repeatedly scrambled, over and over again, to produce an extraordinary range of possible combinations – and hence, able to recognise a near-infinite range of antigens. Then, in a critical process that's still a bit of a mystery, any resulting B-cells that make antibodies that recognise one of your body's own proteins – in other words, antibodies that can attack the body – are invited to self-destruct. Thus, by a process of elimination, you're born with a repertoire of B-cells whose antibody targets are 'not you'. (And if this process isn't 100 per cent completed, it can lead to autoimmune diseases like diabetes or multiple sclerosis.)

Once so formed, each of these unique B-cells then spends its life sitting dormant in your body, like a solitary special snowflake, waiting, waiting… until maybe, one day, a passing dendritic cell presents it with a fragment of an antigen that its antibody is able to recognise. This kicks off a cascade of signals that, ultimately, cause the B-cell to start multiplying rapidly, forming a population of thousands of identical clones, all furiously excreting antibodies into the bloodstream to stick to and neutralise any antigen they encounter. And once the issue has been dealt with, and no more antigen remains, the B-cell then enters a dormant state, ready to reawaken should the infection recur. These so-called memory B-cells are one way you become immune to certain infections, and the basis for how vaccines work.

A quick but important sidebar: in the mid-1970s, researchers started to work out how to artificially generate antibodies against pretty much any antigen they desired. This extraordinary, Nobel-winning feat of biochemical engineering opened up an entire new frontier in medical research and, ultimately, medicine. Because among other uses, these synthetic antibodies – known as monoclonal antibodies – can be used as drugs to target a whole variety of proteins – and, hence, diseases. We'll come back to these antibody drugs later.

OK, that's B-cells. But if you thought *that* was complicated, wait until you hear about the other type of lymphocyte – one that I briefly mentioned in the previous chapter: the T-cell.

Military metaphors can be helpful when talking about the immune system, and if B-cells are archers, launching volleys of highly targeted molecular arrows into the bloodstream, then T-cells are the generals and the foot soldiers.

Key to how T-cells work is a unique protein they bear on their surface, called the T-cell receptor. Just as with antibodies, these are molecular recognition devices, and your body contains a vast number of different T-cells, each bearing a unique receptor. And again similar to B-cells, the vast majority of your body's T-cells lie dormant in your lymph nodes, waiting for an eager dendritic cell to wake them up by presenting them with just the right antigen, in just the right way – and thus trigger them to start multiplying. But unlike B-cells, what happens next is very different.

Once activated, T-cells leave the cosy home of their resident lymph node and migrate through the blood and lymphatic systems to the site of the problem. There, they use their T-cell receptor to look for cells bearing the same antigen they were 'shown' by the dendritic cell that woke them up. Once they find their target, they do one of two things.

Some T-cells, known as 'helper' T-cells, immediately start secreting chemical signals called cytokines. There are hundreds of different cytokines, which all have different effects; which of them a T-cell secretes, and under what circumstances, is still an active area of research. But broadly speaking, you can think of an activated helper T-cell's job as telling other cells what to do — including other immune cells. Hence, you can, for now, consider them the immune army's generals, coordinating the skirmish and dictating tactics. Importantly, they also play a vital role in calling off the assault once the battle is won, and standing down the troops.

The other type of T-cell is the 'killer', or cytotoxic, T-cell, and – from the point of view of our in-built defence against cancer – these are thought to be the most important, vital player. When a killer T-cell finds its target, it unleashes a powerful set of molecular weaponry that punctures the target cell's membrane, triggering it to die by apoptosis. This is cellular hand-to-hand combat – a destructive force so potent that, if not incredibly tightly regulated, can be devastating and lethal. It never ceases to amaze me that our bodies contain within them – within you, within me, right now – a system so powerful that, if unleashed to its full potential, it would literally dissolve you outright within hours. The fact that we don't constantly self-destruct is pretty incredible.

Now, one more thing before we turn back to cancer. I need to discuss, briefly, how the normal cells in your body (including dendritic cells) 'present' antigens on their surface. I think this is the point in my undergraduate lectures where my head finally exploded. It's really, *really* cool.

As your cells go about their business, sitting there, doing their thing, they constantly break down and recycle the proteins they make to do their job. Partly, this is because proteins get old and clapped-out, and are a vital source of amino acids to make new ones. But it's also a vital part of how our immune system works: tiny fragments of these broken-down proteins – called peptide antigens – are also funnelled into a different process. Deep inside the cell, they're mounted on to a specialised protein platform called the major histocompatibility complex (MHC to its friends), which is then ferried to the cell's surface, where the whole thing is exposed to the outside world – and to any passing T-cell. In other words, like a weird needy flasher, every single one of your cells, all day, every day, is constantly exposing its bits to the world, saying, 'Look! I'm normal!'

Now, should some process inside a cell go wrong – say, it becomes infected with a virus, and starts producing foreign, viral proteins – tiny

125

fragments of 'other' start to become incorporated into the cell's MHC proteins, and 'presented' to passing immune cells. Recognising the foreign substance, the T-cell unleashes its lethal payload, killing the problem cell.

Evolution has given us a monstrously powerful weapon, but it's one that comes with a whole slew of safety switches to make sure it never, *ever* fires by mistake, and always only ever fires when the time is right. Many of these safety 'switches' – signals that say, 'Look, I'm normal, don't eat me!' – are proteins on the surface of cells, both immune cells and other cells, that have to be present, or absent, when a T-cell receptor encounters an MHC protein bearing an unusual peptide.

These conceptual switches are called 'immune checkpoints' – and they are absolutely fundamental to understanding how cancer hides itself from the immune system – and how researchers are, gradually, learning how to unmask it.

Let's get into some cancer immunology, and perhaps the greatest (and, paradoxically, hyped) breakthrough in modern medicine: the advent of immunotherapy.

––––––––

Evidence that our immune system plays a crucial role in preventing us getting cancer, and – on occasion – eradicating it from our bodies, has been hiding in plain sight for more than 130 years. The challenge has been working out how to turn these disparate observations into a reliable way to treat patients.

Exhibit one: people with compromised immune systems – such as those with HIV/AIDS, or immunosuppressed transplant patients – are prone to a range of cancers (in fact, studying patterns of cancer incidence was what first alerted researchers to the virus that would turn out to be HIV).

Exhibit two: on the flip side, certain incredibly lucky patients see their cancers just simply disappear – something called 'spontaneous regression', which clever people have estimated to occur in around 1 in every 60,000 to 100,000 people with cancer (and with around 360,000 new cancer cases in the UK every year, it's something worth bearing in mind when reading about the latest 'miracle cure' in the tabloids).

Exhibit three: a related phenomenon known as the 'abscopal effect', in which a patient – often with very advanced cancer – is given radiotherapy to a single tumour (usually to shrink it to relieve the symptoms it causes), and then, miraculously, all the other tumours in their body suddenly disappear, as if a switch were suddenly thrown.

And then there's the smoking gun: Coley's toxin – perhaps the first ever (albeit incredibly crude) cancer immunotherapy.

In the mid-1800s, doctors in Germany noticed that patients' tumours could occasionally shrink after they'd also had a skin infection called erysipelas. By the end of the century, a New York-based doctor called William Coley had developed a method of injecting advanced cancer patients with a cocktail of dead bacteria derived from these skin lesions. Despite a fair few successes – he rather grandiosely claimed to have cured more than 1000 patients – the technique was extremely patchy. And then radiotherapy came along, and Coley's toxin fell out of favour as researchers focused their efforts on that instead.

There was another brief flurry of interest in immune-based therapies to treat cancer in the 1960s and 70s, as various cytokines – the immune system's signalling molecules – were discovered. Perhaps the most notable of these was a cytokine called interferon, part of the body's natural defence against viruses. After a few small trials showed promise, a huge hype-bubble blew up around interferon – a prominent BBC documentary in the early 70s hailed it as the 'new cure'. Alas, as well as only showing marginal benefit in larger trials, the treatment's side effects – florid flu-like symptoms – proved to be too much for many to bear (it turns out that the 'symptoms' of flu are actually caused, in part, by a massive release of interferon). Together, this was enough to halt its development as a mainstream cancer therapy, although it continued to be used as a last resort in a few situations – including, until quite recently, advanced melanoma.

Around the same time, there was a parallel effort to develop so-called cancer vaccines – short, injectable peptides derived from proteins known to be overproduced by cancers. The theory was sound: wake up the patient's immune system by giving them a massive dose of cancer proteins. And in a very small minority of patients, this seemed to work – but not often enough to be worth testing in larger trials.

Another strategy was to genetically modify certain viruses – which were known to reproduce preferentially inside cancer cells – so that they programmed infected cells to release cytokines, thus alerting the immune system to their presence. Again, despite the odd dramatic response, this approach failed too.

Researchers continued to persist with immunotherapy because of those rare dramatic responses – clearly *something* was happening: flickers of seemingly random success, but nothing reliable, and certainly nothing to prove better, overall, than the standard treatments of radiotherapy or ever more sophisticated cocktails of chemotherapy. By the mid-1990s there was another distraction – a new kid on the block: the new generation of drugs like imatinib and vemurafenib, which were designed to target cells with particular faulty genes. Moving into the new millennium, many research organisations – Cancer Research UK among them – began to turn their efforts towards sequencing more and more DNA, convinced the answer to cancer lay within its chaotic genome, and the scrambled genes within.

In retrospect, what was missing was a vital bit of the puzzle, one that was only discovered in the mid-1990s, and which I mentioned earlier – immune checkpoint proteins, the switches on the surface of both immune and non-immune cells that govern whether, in a given scenario, the immune system should fire or not.

It was a discovery that could explain all the disappointing failures. No matter how much cytokine you injected into a patient, or how sophisticated the peptide vaccine, getting the immune system to fire *without also flipping one of the checkpoint switches* meant the approach would be doomed to fail. Nature's tight control of where and when to activate the immune systems had finally been understood – now the field could move forward.

The full heroic story of the discovery of checkpoint proteins, and the subsequent development of powerful cancer treatments known as checkpoint inhibitors, is dealt with beautifully in other books – notably Charles Graeber's excellent *The Breakthrough*[1] – and I won't regurgitate it here. The key thing for our story is that in 2010 – three years before Annabell was diagnosed with melanoma – the first drug designed to target these checkpoint molecules showed promise in a large international trial[2] for patients with advanced melanoma (a cancer type chosen for these initial trials in part because it's one that appears particularly susceptible to immune-related phenomena like spontaneous regression and the abscopal effect).

The drug, ipilimumab, is – like many modern cancer drugs – something called a monoclonal antibody (this is why so many drug names end in -mab; they're **monoclonal antibodies**),* specifically engineered to stick tightly to a particular molecule. In ipilimumab's case, it sticks to an immune checkpoint protein called CTLA-4, found on the surface of T-cells.

CTLA-4 had been discovered by a team of US researchers in the 90s, led by Professor Jim Allison (who'd go on to share a Nobel Prize for this work), and which included a young Sergio Quezada – now at UCL and involved with Zarah's story.

CTLA-4 works a bit like a snooze control on an alarm clock: if it's pressed, it prevents T-cells bearing it from being woken up. Its exact workings are still being scrutinised, but the leading idea is that it affects immune cells in the lymph nodes. Here, dendritic cells present fragments of antigens they've found to the T-cells snoozing there, in an effort to rouse them. But for cancer antigens, for reasons unknown – perhaps because they're too 'self-like' – this interaction isn't normally very strong, a gentle shake rather than a full bellow, and the presence of CTLA-4 on the T-cells stops the antigen-bearing dendritic cells from awakening them.

The ipilimumab antibody appears to work by covering up the CTLA-4 switch, preventing it from being pressed, and allowing the dendritic cells to kick-start the immune system.†

Regardless of the underlying mechanism, the trials were clear: in around 1 in 10 patients with very advanced melanoma, the drug awakened their immune system, causing their tumours to melt away. Many of the patients on the original trials are still alive today – far

---

*You may be wondering: what about the ones that end in -nib? These are **inhib**itors. For example, 'vemurafenib' belongs to a class of drugs called 'raf inhibitors' – hence the '-rafenib' suffix. There is a method, of sorts, to the apparent madness of drug names.

†A brief aside. There's a competing theory that the drug works very differently: it sticks to CTLA-4 molecules on a type of T-cell called a regulatory T-cell, and so performs an antibody's 'natural' role: labelling these cells for destruction by cell-eating macrophages. Regulatory T-cells are involved in damping down or switching off an ongoing immune response, and tumours seem to recruit to their neighbourhood to shield them from immune attack. It will be fascinating to see how this pans out, as it could yield clues to developing more effective immunotherapies.

beyond what would normally be expected. It was a dramatic finding, and in December 2012 – the year before Annabell's diagnosis, and two years before her cancer's spread became rapid and aggressive – it was approved for routine use on the NHS.

But ipilimumab came with a couple of big downsides. The first, as I've said, was that there was – and still is – no way of telling who would respond.

The second was that, far from being a 'gentler' treatment than chemo, ipilimumab's ability to indiscriminately activate the immune system meant it could cause some absolutely horrendous side effects. Although rare, deaths had occurred on the initial trials, as patients' hyperactive immune systems were let loose, causing particularly serious bouts of colitis – an inflammatory bowel condition – and pneumonitis, a similar condition in the lungs. These were manageable with high doses of steroids, but 'ipi' – as it had become known – was no walk in the park. And as with the drug's benefits, it was impossible to tell who might develop the side effects.

When you're dealing with advanced, life-threatening cancer, however, these are all gambles worth considering – particularly given that, unlike chemotherapy and targeted drugs, those who did respond seemed to have what was being described, somewhat euphemistically, as 'long, durable responses'. In other words, they were completely cancer-free. It now seems likely that these people are cured.

And so for Annabell, with her melanoma rapidly on the march, it was a potentially life-saving option.

———

Annabell had her first dose of ipilimumab in February 2015 and, initially, things seemed to go fine. The major downsides were, in fact, psychological.

She recalls: 'Because it was a new thing, they were so concerned about reporting side effects, and I had this long checklist that I had to fill in every day. So I just spent the whole time noting down every small thing, like headaches, rashes, like, everything... I stopped drinking, and I tried to eat really well.'

The plan was for her to receive four doses of the drug, intravenously, three weeks apart, during appointments in Barts Hospital. Meanwhile, she was still going to work, trying to have a regular life, keeping on keeping on.

But worrying about the side effects was taking its toll.

'I was so obsessed by it that I wasn't really, kind of, enjoying life in any way. Which is kind of stupid because I'd had melanoma for more than a year by that point. I was like, well, why wasn't I so bothered about this before?'

Then, after the third dose, things started to slide. 'I started having diarrhoea a lot, and so then they wouldn't give me the fourth dose. But I had a week of steroids and things calmed down a bit, so then they gave the final dose.'

Après ça, le déluge. Two weeks later – just three days after she and James moved in together – her diarrhoea dramatically worsened and she was admitted to hospital with severe colitis, where she'd stay for nearly a month, unable to eat. 'I didn't leave that room once,' she says. James visited her every day. The boxes in their new home remained unpacked.

I remember going to visit her with Zarah – it was the first time we'd been to Barts Cancer Centre, a gleaming new building with a large, spacious atrium full of sad-eyed people in limbo – and I remember how emaciated she was, almost unrecognisable. But I reassured Zarah: Annabell was getting the latest, most cutting-edge treatment, in a modern, new cancer centre – she was in the best possible hands.

But good hands alone aren't enough to hold melanoma back. By August, Annabell's latest scans had shown that, despite the immunotherapy, yet another melanoma had appeared on her leg, and had also started to spread to her liver. She was devastated.

'I was like, what the fuck, I'm trying my hardest on these drugs, and they're not working, and everyone had been so excited, it was the cure, the next big thing. That was hard.'

Over this period, James had started to go to Annabell's appointments with her. Previously, she'd relied on her family – sister Sophie, brother Simon, and her father, Alan, and mother, Sue – the latter of whom was there for every bit of news, good and bad, that Annabell had heard. In particular, she remembers, 'Mum and James were both, kind of, like carers for me.'

The news that the ipilimumab hadn't worked meant it was on to the next thing. Tests on her tumour, carried out months previously, had revealed the presence of a hallmark mutation in the BRAF gene – the one that – supposedly – makes tumours sensitive to the targeted drug vemurafenib. Like ipilimumab, it had recently been made available on the NHS. Her doctors immediately switched her to the drug.

And things continued to deteriorate.

Vemurafenib's principal side effect is a nasty skin rash, and by September, Annabell's skin was in a terrible state. Her temperature spiked, and she was, again, admitted to hospital for a short stay. The team reduced her dose, but upped her steroids, causing her rash-ravaged face to become characteristically puffed up. She remembers that, during one visit to hospital, even her consultant failed to recognise her.

And then, just before Christmas – a glimmer of good news: scans suggested that the disease on her liver had, possibly, begun to shrink. 'It was a weird appointment. James and I were both there, it was, like, two days before Christmas, and I had said we'd had to bring it forward so that we could go away. And the consultant, who wasn't our usual doctor, said, "Make sure you have a really great time, make sure you take this drug, but, you know, have a really good holiday, have a really great Christmas."'

'Have a great holiday.' It's a tell, isn't it?

———

I remember that Christmas vividly. Zarah, Lindsey and I had hired a holiday home in a lovely little Kent village. The plan was for Annabell and James to come down and visit for a few days, before heading off to do family things, and then mine and Zarah's mothers would come down for Christmas itself. And so we had a lovely few days with James and Annabell, jumping in cars and heading over the Channel on the Eurotunnel to do a pre-Christmas booze cruise. The five of us pottered around a small French village, Annabell obviously a bit worn down, anxious, but – as usual – not giving too much away.

After they left, our mothers arrived. And later that night, with both asleep upstairs, Zarah, Lindsey and I got horrendously drunk, and cried, and talked about cancer, and death, and what might happen, and what we could do.

We were all desperately worried about what 2016 might bring for Annabell – and blissfully unaware that there was a second time bomb, ticking gently, literally in our midst.

———

2016 – the year everything went to shit. For Zarah, of course, but also for Annabell. 'This was where it all kicked off,' she told me.

In their first appointment of the New Year, James and Annabell received a body blow. There'd been 'a problem' interpreting the scan from before Christmas. A second look had shown that the spots in her liver hadn't actually shrunk, and there were, in fact, a few small signs that the cancer had spread to her lungs.

The vemurafenib wasn't working. She was running out of options.

In fact, there was only, really, one left: a short course of chemotherapy, followed immediately by a newer immunotherapy drug – pembrolizumab – which had, just two months earlier, been approved for routine use in melanoma.

Pembrolizumab (also known as pembro) is, like ipilimumab (ipi), an antibody-based drug, and similarly targets an immune checkpoint protein on the surface of cells. But it works in a very different way, preventing an interaction between two different checkpoint proteins – one, found on immune cells, is known as PD-1; its partner, produced by other cells in the body, is called PD-L1.

Under normal circumstances, these cells deploy PD-L1 as a sort of white flag, signalling to T-cells that everything's fine and dandy. This is a particularly useful skill, for example, for uninfected and otherwise innocent bystanders at the site of an infection, to stop them getting caught in the cellular crossfire.

Cancer cells, the devious fuckers, frequently evolve the ability to wave their PD-L1 white flag, and this allows them to avoid being zapped by T-cells that have sensed their presence, and are closing in, armed and ready to fire. (The researchers who discovered the PD-1/PD-L1 checkpoint shared the Nobel Prize with the discoverers of CTLA-4.)

Pembrolizumab – along with a host of similar new drugs with equally ridiculous names – sticks fast to the PD-1 checkpoint protein on a T-cell's surface, preventing it from being put to sleep by cancer cells bearing PD-L1. Just as with ipilimumab, trials showed occasional dramatic, long-lasting responses in people with advanced melanoma. Just as with ipilimumab, it only works in a minority of melanoma patients, although about twice as many as with ipi. Just as with ipi, it's very difficult to predict who's going to respond. And just as with ipi, there can be serious side effects, although to a lesser degree. There was no guarantee it would work for Annabell, and a sizeable chance it could put her back in hospital.

But like I said, when you've got advanced cancer, odds are a foreign country.

Before Annabell was to receive this last line of hope, first she would receive three cycles of good old-fashioned combination chemotherapy, with two drugs – a plant alkaloid called paclitaxel and a platinum-based drug called carboplatin. This was because, even when immunotherapy drugs work, they can take a while – sometimes months – to kick the immune system into gear. Quite sensibly, Annabell's doctors wanted to use the chemo to buy time, holding her disease in check long enough for the pembro to work.

It was tough news to take. No one looks forward to chemotherapy. 'Chemo's the bad boy, isn't it? When they start chemo, they don't put a ribbon round it,' Annabell remembered.

Shortly after starting chemo, in early 2016, she went over to Lindsey's to have dinner with her and Zarah, who'd just got back from visiting her sick father in Ireland, and who seemed really keen to meet up.

'So Linds cooked this fancy dinner, and they asked me how things were going with the chemo, and then we went to the living room and sat there for quite a bit, and Zarah told us about her dad.

'And then, while telling us about what had happened with her dad, she started talking about what had happened for her in hospital there. And then she said, "They've diagnosed me with bladder cancer, and it's quite severe".'

Annabell remembers the numbing shock, 'but also I had this weird feeling – this is going to sound like so selfish, given what happened later that I was the lucky one. Because I felt like I was out of the diagnosis stage when everything was horrible – I had this path that I was already on, but my heart was breaking for you and Zarah, because you were at the beginning of this horrible, horrible thing. And I felt lucky to not be back there. I was almost… settled into the process of having cancer, I had chemo, I had options. And James and I just wanted to do everything we could for you both.'

And there you have it. The stories have collided.

But wait. It gets worse. With cancer, it usually does.

After learning of her friend's diagnosis, Annabell's 'lucky feeling' didn't last more than a few more days: right after her first cycle of chemotherapy, she started getting headaches.

At first, she put it down to the chemo. Headaches, after all, had been mentioned as a potential side effect. But then they started to get worse.

'I'd had a few drinks on Saturday night, maybe two glasses of wine – the most I'd had so far during the chemo – but on the Sunday I couldn't get out of bed, my head was throbbing so much. I thought I was tired, or maybe a bit dehydrated from drinking.' She was still working three days a week, so called in sick on Monday. By Tuesday, she could barely get out of bed. On the Wednesday, she and James headed in to Barts for a scheduled appointment with her consultant – who ordered an immediate brain scan.

'Immediate', in NHS terms, meant a three-hour wait. James went back to work while Annabell waited. 'I remember telling him, oh, don't worry, it's just a scan, we never find anything at scans anyway, and then while waiting for the scan I was messaging Zarah, and said, oh, they're making me have the scan today, that's unusual.'

It got more unusual.

'After the scan, they made me sit and wait for the results. They'd never done that before. I remember thinking, this feels weird.'

Annabell waited. And waited. The clock on the waiting room wall ticked up to six o'clock. She was due to meet her mum after the appointment, and was worried about keeping her waiting.

'The ward was winding down for the day, and everyone was walking through there to go home, and I was waiting, just waiting, I didn't know why. And the radiologist came out and said, "We've seen something on your brain. We can't talk to you about it right now. We're trying to get hold of a doctor. Just wait here."'

And no one appeared after that for a very long time. 'I was sat in a corridor where the lights were turned off, and everyone was going through it with their coats on, on their way home, and I was crying because a doctor said they'd seen something in my brain but then just completely disappeared. And I didn't want to talk to James because I didn't want to upset him.

'I don't know how long I waited there, but it felt like a fucking long time. Then, finally, a doctor came down, one that I hadn't seen before – a neurologist. My doctor apparently wasn't around, they couldn't get hold of him.'

The neurologist explained, carefully and clearly, that Annabell had several large tumours in her brain, and needed to have brain surgery, urgently. Her mum and brother, Simon, arrived shortly afterwards, and Annabell gently broke the news to them too.

'That was probably the worst of all days,' she says. Her doctors hadn't mentioned that melanoma could spread to the brain. It was a complete shock.

'I remember around that time various people asking me, like, oh, hasn't anyone mentioned the fact that the brain is the next place it would go to? And they hadn't then. I might have read it somewhere earlier on, but then at that point I also stopped reading about melanoma on the Internet, because I found it so unhelpful, and it just took me to a horrible place. And I stick with that, actually, because regardless of whether it makes me feel informed or not, it does help with my mental health, and I've found that that's helped me along the way.'

Annabell was sent home, accompanied by Sue and Simon, with a sackful of steroids, to help manage what was now 'the worst headache in the world', and told to wait for an appointment for a second scan, to plan the surgery.

Her family were distraught at the wait, and wanted to go private. 'Mum and Simon were so worried, they wanted to get the scan done now, now, now – they wanted to pay. But I remember being weirdly calm about it.' She remembers her sister, Sophie, saying later on how odd she found it that Annabell was so... not 'happy', but was joking about it. 'I think it's just sometimes, at those points you just snap into this kind of survival state.'

A few days passed. Annabell and James tried to be normal. 'We went to Stoke Newington, we had lunch, my brother came and met us, we looked at some vintage shops, we bought coffee cups,' she recalls. 'I remember we were sat in a café, and my brother was trying to talk about calling people to get a scan, and me and James were just sort of laughing. We were just like, well, the nurse has called, and they still didn't have a date.

'But then, on Friday, Lindsey had come round for lunch, and another neurologist called and said, "You need to come to A&E. We don't think you're safe to be at home." Apparently, the positioning of the tumours, and the potential inflammation, meant I was at extremely high risk of having a stroke or a seizure.'

Lindsey helped her pack and they headed to the Royal London, where Annabell spent the weekend in a hospital bed, accompanied by James and Sophie. The operation was scheduled for the following Tuesday.

The day before, her doctors talked her through what it might entail.

'Because of the position where they were, right in the back of my head, and because the main one was quite big, about 5 centimetres, and because the inflammation was touching my spine, there were lots of risks that they were talking about. But the one that stuck with me was that I might be paralysed. I could wake up from that surgery and not be able to move.'

She was still, at this point, remarkably positive about the outlook.

'I wasn't worried about dying then. I was sure I wasn't going to die from that surgery or the brain tumours. Instead, I thought that things were going to be very different. Like, I don't know how, but when I wake up, things are going to be completely different.' She remembers emailing her brother and sister the morning of the operation. 'I was like, I know I'm not going to die this time, you can't get rid of me that easily.'

In the end, the operation went well, and seemed to have removed the tumours. But to reach them, the surgeon had needed to cut through the muscles round the top of her spine, and it was a week before she'd be able to walk properly – and even then, she needed a walking stick for nearly two months as she slowly recovered.

But two weeks after the operation, it was time for the last roll of the dice.

At the beginning of March, Annabell had her first dose of pembrolizumab immunotherapy.

Although she'd been thrown a lifeline, things for Annabell started getting pretty bleak psychologically.

'Since I hadn't responded to other drugs, I was worried about not responding. The doctors were very concerned that my colitis would flare up again. I was taking quite a lot of steroids to reduce the inflammation from the brain surgery, and I was trying to come off those, but every time I reduced the dose I got more headaches, or more sick.

'But also I knew I needed something, and nothing else had worked. There weren't any other options at that point.

'It was around that time when I suddenly started worrying about dying. I even stopped walking with a stick, because I thought, well, if I'm going to die, then I don't want to be remembered like this, hobbling around with a stick.'

Around this time, she and James had a surreal conversation with her consultant.

'I've never been able to get my head around it. He said, "Your GP's called me up asking what's happened, because she's just been through your notes. She's asked me what your prognosis was, and whether I've told you."

'And then he asked me, "Well, do you want to know your prognosis?"'

James and Annabell were completely thrown.

'So we asked him: what's the prognosis?

'And this is what he said: "If it wasn't for modern medicine, you wouldn't be alive right now, so I don't really know what your prognosis is."'

He also – to James and Annabell's mutual amazement – brought up the story of former US President Jimmy Carter, whose dramatic, positive response to pembrolizumab had made headlines around the world.

This talk of elderly American presidents and unknown prognoses left Annabell feeling perplexed. 'I had no way to interpret what he was saying, other than "it's a surprise I'm still alive". But I became consumed with worrying I was going to die any minute, basically. I just started thinking, my life's going to be over very soon.'

And then, as if it were even possible on top of all that: another gut punch. A follow-up scan in mid-April, after just her second dose of pembro, revealed yet more tumours in her brain. Three of them.

Her doctors debated what to do.

The neurosurgeon felt that the largest was too big to remove safely, the risks too great, the benefits too small. He really didn't want to operate.

Her oncologist, on the other hand, wanted to buy her time for the pembrolizumab to kick in. There were rumours of a row. If his colleague were to remove the largest tumour, he argued, the other two could be zapped with radiotherapy to slow their growth, and give the pembro a chance to kick-start Annabell's immune system. For him, three was the magic number: the number of doses of pembro that studies suggested were needed to properly light the fire in Annabell's immune system.

The cynical surgeon versus the optimistic oncologist. It's a debate played out over and over throughout the history of cancer medicine. The former acutely aware of the fragility of the human body, wary of the well-worn path of hype and disappointment that's been trodden, over and over, in cancer drug discovery. The latter convinced that this time, it might be different; this drug might be the one.

On this occasion, the oncologist's arguments won the day.

They decided to operate.

Unlike last time, however, for Annabell there was no sunny optimism, no conviction everything would be OK. Nothing had worked so far. Numbly, and despite the huge risk that she might not wake up, or might wake up profoundly disabled, or mute, she consented to her second round of brain surgery. It was this or nothing.

A few days later, in the corridor outside the operating theatre, James was waiting with Annabell. It was time for the operation. Through the tears, they said goodbye, knowing it might be the last word they spoke to each other.

I remember getting a text from Zarah – who was, at the time, in Cork vising her family, but worried out of her mind about her friend – that Annabell's surgery had gone OK. That she was awake, and talking. I was in New Orleans at the time, deep in the bowels of an enormous conference centre, surrounded by some of the leading minds in contemporary cancer research, and being bombarded by graphs and charts and data showing that the tide was turning, that cancer was controllable, that cures were on the way.

And I remember thinking, then, that all the hope and optimism we had was being validated, that Zarah, too, was going to be OK; that our faith in modern medicine was justified. Annabell's story was bleak, and full of the most convoluted, painful twists and turns. But she was still there, still alive, still in with a chance.

To paraphrase a quote: You can take the despair.

It's the hope that really gets you.

———————

Brain surgery out of the way, it was now time for Annabell to complete what had become a bizarre game of cancer treatment bingo. Having had surgery, electrochemotherapy, immunotherapy, targeted therapy, chemotherapy, brain surgery, and more immunotherapy, Annabell went for the 'full house' – a series of doses of radiotherapy, targeted as precisely as possible to the remaining tumours in her brain.

Then, basically, it was back home. To sit and wait. And hope. And cross everything.

And finally, at long last – after everything that'd been thrown at her, after all the twists and turns and hope and devastation and all the rest – gradually, the storm clouds began to part.

The first scan after the radiotherapy showed encouraging signs: the tumours in her brain had started to recede; elsewhere, her disease looked stable.

More good news soon after: a subsequent scan, in September, showed that the tumours in her liver and lung had also started to shrink.

It looked, touch wood, like the pembrolizumab might be working. Everyone was over the moon. Everyone except Annabell, who didn't want to let her guard down just yet.

'That was probably the first point where it was like, OK, this is actually... things are actually... changing. That means I can keep on this drug, that means it's actually working. But I was still on steroids, still having to take the drug, still having regular scans... and I guess I still thought I was going to die.'

She remembers feeling exceptionally cautious – particularly since everyone else seemed so delighted.

'I couldn't think about the next year, at all. I didn't really believe in "next year". But I can really vividly remember what other people thought about it.'

It was, however, a turning point. Annabell would keep taking pembrolizumab, every three weeks, until... well, nobody seemed terribly clear on that point.

Zarah and I were, of course, delighted – for Annabell, and for James too. And also, a little selfishly, really pleased that the hype around immunotherapy seemed justified – we were pinning rather a lot of our own hopes on these magic antibodies, and to hear that the treatment was working for Annabell was a much-needed boost for us too. But I must also confess, the small dank corner of my brain where my anxieties and insecurities live was sending out some worrying messages. Two friends, both with advanced cancer? What were the chances? And both pinning their hopes on immunotherapy, a treatment that fails to work more often than it succeeds? And one of them seems to be responding? What, that corner of my brain said, were the chances that both of them would?

I suppressed that thought immediately – after all, it had no rational basis. There was nothing about what went on in Annabell's body that affected what might go on in Zarah's. It was just statistics.

Just statistics.

But wait. We've got ahead of ourselves now. Let's rewind slightly. We'll pick up Annabell's story, and how she fared on the immunotherapy, a bit later. We need to get back to Zarah's timeline now, in July, just after we'd had our own good news, that her chemo seemed to be working, as we were gearing up for a much-needed break.

5

What next?

VII: Rebirth

Scene: The battle-ravaged lining of the bladder. A scarred, bloody vista of inflamed tissue and slowly leaking capillaries, infused with a harsh, alien toxin.

Zoom in: Patrolling immune cells squeeze themselves through the debris-strewn layers of cells, their molecular weaponry poised to fire at the slightest sign of trouble. Cell by cell, they check for hallmarks of their foe, scanning the surface of each one, occasionally unleashing a powerful stream of perforating toxins when a rogue cell is detected. But increasingly, in the aftermath of the epic battle, all appears quiet.

Watch: Slowly, as the concentration of the toxin drops, the tissue becomes home once more to thousands of wobbly macrophages, hoovering up the cellular debris left over from the battle, while secreting molecular signals to calm things down, and gently begin the healing process.

In response to these signals, new blood vessels begin to form, branching out, suffusing the tissue with nutrients. Damaged capillaries are repaired. The bleeding slowly stops. The immune cells, becalmed, gradually holster their weapons. The whole system attempts, gradually, to return to something approaching 'normal'.

But it is a false dawn.

Stop. Shift focus: Deep within the slowly healing tissue, something stirs. A small clump of cells that has remained somehow hidden from the immune cells' scrutiny. Unlike their multitude of now-deceased siblings, these rare cells – each a distant descendant of that rogue mother cell – are different, their internal wiring subtly scrambled in a different way, unable to commit suicide, locked in suspended animation, doomed to continue their mindless existence, waiting for conditions to improve.

Now is their moment.

As the toxin's levels recede, these resistant mutants' ragged, disordered, chaotic chromosomes shudder into life, condensing, lining up as best they can on the cells' central skeleton once more. The cells repeatedly cleave in two, into four, into eight, into sixteen – exponentially growing once more, undetected, still no smaller than a pinprick.

Zoom out. Shift focus. Zoom in again. Another microscopic mass of cells, and another. Hundreds, thousands, of tiny quiescent clumps. All have been similarly dormant, similarly cloaked, an underground resistance movement, weathering the onslaught. All are now buzzing with activity, released from stasis. Bursting into morbid life once again.

Slowly, the now resistant monster marshals its forces, and begins to rebuild anew.

July had arrived, and with it some absolutely glorious weather. Proper, balmy, un-British, 30-plus-degree heat. The sort we Brits pretend only happens for like a day a year – this stuff lasted weeks. It felt like a sign. We got ready for the first of a couple of mini-holidays. Tina the tumour, being Tina, had another grumble: just before we were due to depart, Zarah's bladder infection flared up again. More antibiotics, a couple more frustrating nights in Westmoreland Hospital for a quick scan to check her stent wasn't full of gunk. But eventually the doctors were happy that everything was OK – we were good to travel. So off we trotted, armed with a sack of hardcore antibiotics ('pipe cleaner', we overheard one of the nurses call it), and a cornucopia of analgesics.

We borrowed a car, and first drove back to my mum's friend's cottage in the Chilterns. Unlike last time – a chilly early spring, with bluebells and open fires and snuggly pubs – this time it was shorts, T-shirts, G&Ts by the pool, BBQs in the evening. A few close friends came with us; a couple we'd met while travelling swung by, as did my mum. Lounging by a pool in swimming costumes, booze in hand, *in the UK* was a first for us all. Happy, happy memories. You don't look like you have cancer. After five glorious days in the English countryside, we got ready to pack up and drive back to London, thence on to a flight to Barcelona. Tina, of course, kept popping her head in to remind us of our febrile existence – just before we left the cottage, Zarah passed another massive blood clot in the loo, and the pain in her lower back suddenly began to spike through the painkillers. I remember crouching in the doorway of a shop in a quaint little English village, chatting anxiously to Dr Mark Linch at UCLH, asking if it was still sensible to fly to Spain. He reassured me it'd be fine, and if anything went wrong, the Spanish medical system was top-notch – and we were just a short plane journey from UCLH, should we need to get back quickly.

So off to Barcelona we went. More fun was had – hanging out in bars, scoffing tapas, staying up late with old friends, enormous goldfish-bowl G&Ts, and having long, lazy lie-ins as the sun streamed through the bay windows of our apartment. We went for a day trip to the beach – 'bitches in Sitges', we joked – took in an incomprehensible Catalan drag show. More happy memories. But compared to previous travelling adventures, the pace of our life had slowed, the dynamic forever changed by Zarah's disease – she was still easily tired, the pain never too far away. We planned our pottering around the now routine schedule of painkillers. Tina was still with us, even if she was keeping relatively quiet.

And then, with unnerving timing, as we stepped on to the coach to the airport, Zarah's back pain suddenly worsened. 'That's yer lot for now,' Tina seemed to be saying. We scrabbled around in my backpack for the morphine. By the time we landed, Zarah was in agony, and neither paracetamol nor morphine could hold it in check. So, straight from the airport, we took the now well-trodden path up to the 14th floor of UCLH for another round of scans and tests to make sure nothing was seriously amiss. People talk about 'post-holiday blues' – well, it doesn't get more crashingly depressing than going from Stansted's baggage reclaim hall to an oncology ward. We were back where we began.

Three more nights in hospital. More scans. More tests. Still no sign of an infection. The best guess, from all the recent evidence, was that Zarah's swollen, inflamed, fluid-filled lymph nodes were pressing against nerves in her abdomen. There was a brief discussion, once again, of some radiotherapy to try to shrink things down.

But radiotherapy brought complications with it, and not just in terms of side effects. There was a whole new consideration weighing on our minds: just before our holiday, we had our first appointment with a team at Barts to discuss immunotherapy trials – specifically, how to get Zarah on to one as soon as possible.

It had been weird, going to a different hospital, part of a different NHS Trust. Things were the same but different. A different waiting area. A new receptionist. The same crap Wi-Fi and crap coffee. A different automated voice in the elevator. The same ashen-faced look on the faces of the patients waiting for their appointments.

After a nervous wait, they'd called Zarah's name, and we'd walked down a cramped corridor and into the oncologist's office, where we met Professor Tom Powles for the first time. He's an extraordinary man, Tom. Much younger than we were expecting. Intense. Caring. Thoughtful. A pair of jeans, a roll-neck jumper and a jacket. You'd almost describe him as cool. He has a habit of breaking off in mid-sentence, removing his glasses, looking down at the floor while pinching the bridge of his nose, as if consulting a giant, comprehensive oncology textbook that he carries around in his head.

Right after her last dose of chemo, Zarah had been referred from UCLH over to his team at Barts (although Ursula's team, being her 'primary' team, would be kept abreast of her progress, and on hand if we had any questions).

Leaning forward in his chair, attention fixed intensely on Zarah, Tom ran us through the current situation regarding Barts' immunotherapy trials. Right at that exact moment, there wasn't anything open – but his team were in the middle of getting several new studies off the ground, all of which Zarah might be suitable for.

There were three main options, all of which involved a new antibody-based checkpoint immunotherapy drug called durvalumab. The drug works in a similar way to the pembrolizumab that Annabell was then taking, but differs slightly: the antibody targets the opposite part of the molecular 'handshake' – the PD-L1 on the surface of the cancer cells, rather than the PD-1 on the immune cells.

The first possibility was what's known as a 'maintenance' trial, and was going to recruit people with bladder cancer who'd responded to chemo, and whose disease was now under control (i.e. Zarah's situation at that exact moment). It was a 'randomised' trial – participants would be selected to get either an intravenous infusion of durvalumab, or of a saline placebo, every three weeks. And this would continue until their disease started to grow again. The main aim was to see if immunotherapy would increase the amount of time before cancer started growing again.

The second option was a trial testing a combination of durvalumab and a second tongue-twister of an immuno drug called tremelimumab (which works very similarly to the CTLA-4-targeting ipilimumab). Unlike the previous trial, Zarah would only be eligible for this one if her cancer had started growing again. But unlike the first option, on this trial everyone would get the drug combo. The main aim of this trial, Tom said, was to assess the safety of the drug combo, rather than comparing it to another treatment.

The third trial was a combination of durvalumab with one of a variety of 'targeted' drugs – the ones we discussed back in chapter 2, designed to work in tumours that carry specific genetic faults. This trial, too, was only open to patients whose disease had started growing again after chemo. All patients would get durvalumab, but those with specific gene faults would also get a targeted drug. Similar to the second option, the main aim here was to test the relative safety of the drug combos compared to the immunotherapy on its own.

After he'd finished outlining them, we discussed the options with Tom. I say 'we' – despite his best efforts to keep Zarah in the conversation, this now felt like a direct conversation between Tom and I; our language lapsed into scientific jargon and I fired all sorts of questions at him. I'd immediately grasped the science, I'd been to the conferences, I'd seen some of the preliminary data from other, similar trials. Zarah was, as always, content to let me, her nerdy science geek boyfriend, get stuck in. Later, in our living room, I'd go over it all with her again anyway. I guess some people might call this 'mansplaining'. Those people can fuck off.

The obvious choice – the first trial – had a big drawback: it could result in Zarah getting a saline placebo instead of a potentially effective drug; on top of this, if it didn't work, it could potentially rule out further trials down the line. Plus, it would mean going straight into another round of treatment, possibly for a long time, right after finishing chemo. But we had more holidays to go on.

The second option was really interesting. Although it would be the first time this combo of immunotherapy drugs has been tested in bladder cancer, when a similar combo had been tried in melanoma and lung cancer, it led to a substantial boost in the proportion of patients who responded. But it also carried with it a greater risk of some pretty serious side effects. And there was no guarantee that the drugs would work as well on bladder cancer as they would in these other cancers. (And Tom dropped some hints that he wasn't terribly optimistic that they would.)

The third option was, to my mind, the most intriguing. I knew from writing about it at work that combining targeted drugs with immunotherapy seemed, in some people, to produce really good responses compared to either on their own. But to get any of the combos would mean Zarah's tumour would need to carry one of three or four specific aberrations (Tom was still discussing with the drug company, AstraZeneca, exactly which targeted drugs would be options in the initial phase of the trial). I made a mental note to call Charlie Swanton and see what his team knew about the mutations in Zarah's bladder.

But the kicker with both the second and third options was that, as you might have spotted, we'd have to wait for Zarah's disease to start growing again. It was a horrible Catch-22. Go straight into more treatment and forsake our holidays, or wait for things to go downhill.

Regardless, it was all hypothetical at this point – none of the trials were yet open and recruiting patients. We'd have to wait several weeks for the necessary paperwork, ethical approval, and other bureaucratic ephemera to be completed.

So, along with the pain, the worry, and the stress, these decisions, these options, had been swirling around our heads as we'd been relaxing in the countryside, and pottering around the streets of Barcelona. It was quite an extraordinary psychological state to be in – waiting for NHS bureaucracy, and potentially catastrophic new tumour growth, to determine our future. And even then, which trial should we go for?

Weeks later, back from our mini-break, with Zarah discharged from her post-holiday stint in UCLH, this question began to resolve itself. We headed in for another appointment at Barts with Tom, to find out the lie of the land with respect to clinical trials. While we'd been away, he had been busy. The third option – the trial of immunotherapy in combination with targeted drugs – was about to open (for reasons unknown, the other two were lagging behind). As is so often the case, the trial had a slightly whacky pseudo-acronymic name: BISCAY. It was being funded by AstraZeneca. And for Zarah to be eligible for it, she'd have to meet a variety of criteria (we'll come to these later) – and have another biopsy on her tumour to test it for the presence or absence of various mutations. As far as progression was concerned, Tom felt that the uncertainty over Zarah's scans meant that she might fulfil the criteria as it could mean her tumour was, perhaps, progressing – even though he went to great pains to reassure us that this was a bureaucratic rather than medical view. Would we like to enrol? Whatever happened, even if Zarah's biopsy sample tested negative for the mutations that would grant her access to the drug combo, she'd still get the immunotherapy drug, durvalumab.

If we could have, we'd have bitten his hand off.

The following weekend, we went camping, at a music festival, with a whole host of our friends. It was absolutely glorious weather. Zarah was by now in a lot of pain, which was usually well controlled, but would occasionally break through into shuddering, groaning agony. She needed to stay seated if she could. She'd also started to develop lymphoedema in her right leg, which was impeding her movement a bit. But knowing that the trial would soon be opening, that she'd soon be given a next-generation, high-tech immunotherapy that had a significant chance of helping her, as it was helping Annabell, gave her the mental strength to keep going. The festival theme was: 'Who did you want to be when you grew up?' She and Lindsey dressed as Patsy and Edina from *Absolutely Fabulous*.

They looked amazing. You'd probably guess she was ill, but you'd never guess she had cancer.

The next chapter in our story is the one where, looking back, the wheels on the bus started to wobble, if not detach entirely. Yet so hopeful were we, so focused on the upsides and the positives – the trial, the response to chemo – and on getting through the day-to-day, we didn't really twig at the time. It just seemed to be yet more ups and downs, more loops of the roller-coaster. In reality, it was the beginning of the final descent. Hindsight is powerful. It's also painful.

Round about this time, Zarah was put in touch with the palliative care services provided by our local hospice.

St Joseph's, situated 10 minutes' walk from our flat, on Hackney's busy Mare Street, is arguably the oldest hospice in the UK. I must have gone past it on the bus a hundred times and never noticed it. (I still go past it on the bus, but now I look the other way.) It's an incredibly peaceful, calm place. And yet, for many – including me – a deeply sad one.

Up until this point, neither of us really knew what a 'hospice' was, other than somewhere you go to die – I guess unless you've needed one, or a relative or friend has, you never really need to know. As we were to discover, hospices do so much more than provide a peaceful space to slip away – they're staffed by wonderful, compassionate medical teams, and offer a whole slew of services in addition to medical care. Counselling, massage, support groups, out-of-hours home care... so much useful stuff when you're living with a chronic illness. But our first real engagement with them was in managing – palliating – Zarah's pain.

Palliative care is a loaded term, being synonymous in most people's minds with the much starker phrase, 'end of life' care. The World Health Organization somewhat wordily defines it as 'an approach that improves the quality of life of patients and their families facing the problem associated with life-threatening illness, through the prevention and relief of suffering by means of early identification and impeccable assessment and treatment of pain and other problems, physical, psychosocial and spiritual'. In other words, it's about helping you live, not helping you die.

But when you've got advanced cancer, and someone offers you 'palliative' care, your first thought is, hang on, are you saying I'm dying? Zarah *freaked* when the phrase was first mentioned – I guess because it punctured our carefully constructed bubble of positivity. But once she'd met the staff at St Joseph's, had her first counselling session, a couple of massages, and had a phone consultation with one of the nurses, we both realised that this was a place to be embraced, not feared.

By early August – as we were signing Zarah up for the BISCAY trial and coming to terms with life post-chemo – St Joe's had already taken over responsibility for her 'pain plan'. This now involved regular painkillers every morning and evening – slow-release morphine and pregabalin tablets – along with paracetamol as and when, and sticky syringe-fulls of oral morphine, should things get shaky. This was a lot of opiates, so she was becoming pretty bunged up, gastrically speaking, so she'd also take regular laxatives, morning and evening. Oh, and diazepam to help her sleep. This added up to a complex schedule of pills and potions, which we managed with the help of a mobile app, and a small yellow capsule from a Kinder Surprise chocolate egg (you know, the ones the toys come in), which would rattle around her handbag with the next cocktail of drugs in, ready for her next scheduled doses. The main drug stash lived in our living room – a black cardboard Ikea box we dubbed 'the cancer box', which also contained various notes and leaflets from different bits of the NHS. It was hard to keep track of all of this – I took on the role of drug minder, syncing the app on her phone with a similar one on mine, so I'd get alerts should she miss a dose (which, given the effect of said cocktail of painkillers on her memory, she frequently did).

Ironically, given this cocktail of super-strength analgesia, the toughest thing to manage was the paracetamol, which, it must be said, is possibly the most underrated painkiller ever discovered. The problem was this: you can take paracetamol four times a day, every four hours. But that only spans a 16-hour period – 8 short of a full 24-hour day. Zarah's back pain was now becoming so serious that it would start to break through after about three and a half hours – keeping track of when the next paracetamol was due, yet trying to space things out to get through a whole day, became a daily struggle. All sorts of tactics were employed – bridging the gaps with ibuprofen or oral morphine; timing bedtime so things would wear off as a diazepam kicked in; taking half a paracetamol instead of a whole one… it was a daily, constant focus. Of course, being Team Twat, we managed the whole thing with good humour and a lot of jokes (Zarah's jitters, if and when the painkillers started to wear off, we dubbed 'pre-gabbaling'; when laxatives kicked in, she'd be 'putting the anal into analgesia'). But frankly, it was fucking awful. Occasionally she'd wake up in the middle of the night in agony, confused, unable to think straight. I'd wake too, consult the drug app, work out what she could take, and administer it and hold her while she floated back to sleep. I confess to sneaking a little oral morphine too, more than once, to get back to sleep, or calm me down after I'd spent half an hour gently rubbing her back as the opiates kicked in, the shaking subsided and she drifted back off.

So, that was our daily grind. But one Friday in mid-August, even this carefully constructed routine was failing to manage her back pain. The small of her back, in particular, was painful to touch. We called St Joe's, and organised a home visit from one of the consultants – the wonderful, kind Dr Maggie, who had the demeanour of a stereotypical Irish Catholic nun, but one with ninja-like skills in caring for people with life-threatening illnesses. In our living room, Maggie gave Zarah a thorough examination, including the reflexes in her feet and arms. Something wasn't quite right. Zarah's foot reflex was a bit sluggish. Concerned, Maggie phoned the Royal London to book Zarah in for an MRI scan. We were reluctant to go. Surely we could just up the painkillers? Patiently, Maggie explained the concept of spinal cord compression. Growing tumours near the spine can press down on the nerves inside. Untreated, this can lead to paralysis. It probably wasn't cord compression, but it needed to be ruled out, urgently.

Once again, we packed an overnight bag, and called a cab to take us to the Royal London's A&E department, where they'd be waiting for us.

I said earlier that if you're a cancer patient with a temperature, you get a speedy pass through A&E. But that was NOTHING compared to what happened when we arrived at reception and uttered the phrase 'spinal cord compression'. The receptionist's demeanour changed instantly. Zarah was put in a wheelchair and whisked through to a bed on the urology ward almost immediately, where we waited patiently for the MRI scan.

And waited.

And then everything went to shit.

A few weeks previously, Zarah had had a biopsy to assess her eligibility for the BISCAY trial. This was almost completely unnoteworthy – she'd gone into Barts in the morning, had a CT scan to map out the tumour, then they'd stuck what was effectively a tiny little apple corer through her lower abdomen into her bladder to remove a few 'cores' of tumour tissue. (We'd had the foresight to let the research team know this was going on, so they could get a sample for their studies too.)

Up in the urology department at The London, in preparation for the MRI scan of her spine, the doctors looked at the CT scans taken during Zarah's biopsy and compared them to the scan she had at the end of chemo. They did not like what they saw. There was something new on the scan.

The way this news was delivered to Zarah, by a couple of unfamiliar oncologists, in an unfamiliar ward, was a model of how NOT to treat patients. 'It looks like the cancer has spread to her spine,' said one. 'Really? I don't think we can say that till the MRI results come back.' IN FRONT OF ZARAH, two doctors discussed whether her cancer was rapidly progressing. I wasn't there at the time, but when a tearful, devastated Zarah phoned me, I headed to her bedside like a flash.

Even more appallingly, we had to wait a further 36 hours for the MRI scanner to become available. Royal London Hospital has one of the busiest A&E wards in Europe. It was the weekend. Sure, there were people who needed a scan more urgently – traffic accident victims, intensive care patients – but to drop a bombshell like 'you might have cancer in your spine' then leave a patient hanging for nearly two days is unforgivable. I've long debated whether to make a formal complaint about this, but, well, other stuff happened.

Zarah finally had an MRI scan on Sunday afternoon, at which point she was transferred in an ambulance from the Royal London urology department to a room on Ward 5A of Barts Cancer Centre, while the scan was looked at by a range of experts. We were still in limbo, in another unfamiliar ward. Zarah was instructed to lie flat and not get out of bed. If she needed to pee, they'd bring her a pan. We weren't allowed to raise the bed above a certain angle. We cried a lot, that afternoon.

Late that night, a young doctor came to give us the results of the MRI scan. We'd expected clarity. We got more uncertainty. According to the text-only radiology report, there was 'extensive involvement of multiple vertebrae' – in plain English, there was cancer in lots of different bits of Zarah's spinal column. 'How many? Where?' we asked. The doctor didn't know – all she had to go on was the terse paragraph of text sent over from the Royal London. We asked to see the scans. The doctor promised to see what she could do.

We cried some more. We were devastated. A mere six weeks after the end of her chemotherapy, Zarah's 'stable' cancer was no longer stable. Tina was on the march.

Zarah wasn't to emerge from Ward 5A for nearly five weeks. That room – thankfully, a private one, with its own bathroom, a fridge, and a view of the whole of North London – became home from home. I emailed my managers at Cancer Research UK to let them know the situation – I wouldn't be in for the foreseeable future. Almost every morning, I'd wake up and cycle or get the Tube over to Barts, and spend the days at her bedside. Her colleagues sent huge bouquets of flowers. Lindsey popped to Argos and bought Zarah a fan (oncology wards are warm places to be, especially in the middle of summer). Our wonderful friend Billy loaded up his tablet computer with several seasons of *RuPaul's Drag Race* and lent it to her indefinitely. Others would swing by and deliver smuggled cans of gin and tonic or other illicit treats (illicit from the point of view of an oncology ward – don't worry, we weren't *that* daft).

In the face of this almost overwhelming kindness and support, we slowly absorbed the new diagnosis – cancer in the spine, possibly the WORST place it can spread to (although 'where's the worst site of metastasis?' is a pretty sick game of Top Trumps to play). There were some crumbs of solace – although the cancer had reached her spine, the spectre of spinal cord compression had been ruled out by further scans. Zarah was now free, in theory, to sit up, to get out of bed and move around. But this new freedom was a false one – her pain was still acute and angry. She was largely immobile.

Tom, meanwhile, had been busy on two fronts: investigating what, exactly, was going on with Zarah's cancer, and getting things ready for her to start on the BISCAY trial.

On the first front, things weren't terribly encouraging. Further scans and blood tests showed that Tina was, in Tom's words, 'more active than I'm comfortable with'. He was desperate to act, but exactly what course of action was still being discussed. There was the possibility of radiotherapy, but the entrance criteria for the BISCAY trial were strict, and having prior radiotherapy could throw a spanner in the works. The other option was aggressive chemotherapy – less problematic for getting on the trial, but of questionable effectiveness. To this day, in terms of extending life, no trial has proven a clear benefit of secondary chemo in bladder cancer once the first drugs have failed. But some patients on these trials did benefit in that their symptoms improved. It might be better than nothing. We hung around in limbo, while behind the scenes a whole slew of experts were consulted. The clock was ticking.

And things weren't much more encouraging with the trial, either. There were two problems here: the first was bureaucratic. AstraZeneca hadn't yet processed Zarah's biopsy sample, so she hadn't been formally assigned to any of the different arms of the trial. But worse: as per the protocol for treating suspected spinal cord compression, the doctors at the Royal London had given Zarah a whopping dose of steroids – and the entrance criteria for the trial dictated that participants could not begin immunotherapy treatment within 28 days of taking steroids. So even if the biopsy results came back tomorrow, Zarah would have to wait until this period was up – and this was weeks away. Tom's frustration with this was evident, as was our distress.

Given the (un)necessary hold-ups with the trial, and with Tina awake and active, Tom felt he needed to act to put a lid on things. On 27 August, Zarah was given an intravenous infusion of two new chemo drugs: paclitaxel and carboplatin. 'This is the grown-up stuff,' Tom said. Among many horrible side effects, the thing we'd dreaded back in January would now happen: Zarah would lose her platinum blonde hair.

It wasn't a decision we took lightly. For starters, Tom – one of the world's top bladder cancer oncologists – thought it was worth it on balance. I was less convinced, so I phoned a friend. More specifically, I phoned Charlie Swanton.

He was on holiday at the time, in Spain, and was driving around the countryside, the signal dropping in and out. On speakerphone, I briefed him on the current situation. What would he do if one of his lung cancer patients was in a similar situation?

'I don't treat bladder cancer, Henners, but if I had a lung cancer patient in this situation, I'd go for the chemo. And if that's what Tom's recommending, I say go with it.' Charlie signed off with some words of sympathy that further put my mind at rest.

So, more chemo it was. Of course, we tried to make light of it. A running joke between us, since we first met, was that Zarah's bleach-blonde hair would, on occasion, style itself into something bearing a striking resemblance to that of the UK's infamous dead pederast, Jimmy Savile. And paclitaxel chemotherapy is one of the plant alkaloids, a chemical first isolated from the needles of a well-known coniferous tree.

So, naturally, we referred to Zarah's second bout of chemotherapy as 'Operation Yewtree'.

I want to dwell for a minute on those weeks on Ward 5A of Barts Cancer Centre, because over the whole period of Zarah's illness, we never received such incredible, cheerful, compassionate care as we did from the staff on that ward. They were, in the truest sense of the word, a team. Danny, the ward manager – a short, cheerful, bespectacled, slightly portly man – introduced himself personally the day after Zarah was admitted. While she was bed-bound, he'd muck in with the rest of the team in changing her sheets – a complex process involving four people lifting various bits of my girlfriend up, removing old sheets and slipping new ones underneath – or helping her with her bedpan. Many of the nurses were clearly good friends outside of the ward. When shifts changed, the incoming staff would invariably be fully up to speed with Zarah's current situation. We knew everyone by their first name, and they knew ours. The day Lindsey arrived with the Argos-bought fan, one of the porters dashed off to find her a screwdriver and helped her assemble it. Whenever I arrived each morning, I'd usually find one of the nurses chatting away to Zarah during their break. Even her now weekly enemas were delivered with good cheer and good humour, despite the frankly horrendous smell.

So too it was with Tom's oncology team – Alison, Fiona, Matt and Peter. They felt like friends. Friends who really cared about my girlfriend.

Yes, Ward 5A was proper care, delivered by expert staff, consistently, for more than a month, against the most desperate of backgrounds. True, wherever she was treated, Zarah would *always* get on with her nurses. And although medical professionals will (and do) *strenuously* deny it, I think it's a fair observation that a beautiful 37-year-old affected by something as awful as stage 4 bladder cancer will always elicit a certain extra degree of sympathy, simply from the tragic rarity of such a condition in one so young. But those factors aside, there was something magical about 5A: an undefinable quality that you only get with a motivated team who all have each other's backs. Obviously, you're never 'lucky' to have to spend five weeks on a cancer ward, but we were lucky to wind up on 5A. I'm still in touch with some of the staff there. They still remember Zarah with an affection that breaks my heart.

There was now so much going on with Zarah's condition that it's hard to write coherently about it. The chemo did what several months of laxatives failed to do, and gave her the chronic shits. Her pain was still persistent. She could barely walk. The lymph node in her right groin was angry and swollen. And her legs – particularly her right leg – were slowly getting larger, as the lymphoedema became more serious. Oh, we'll talk more, much more, about the lymphoedema later – it's one of the few aspects of Zarah's story that I'm still genuinely angry about. For now, all you need to know is that one of Zarah's legs was about 50 per cent larger than the other, further affecting her ability to walk.

August turned to September, and the leaves started falling off the trees. Fittingly, it was also autumn for Zarah's hair. Slowly at first, then in big clumps, her bright, bleach-blonde hair – for so many years her most striking feature, one our friends had used to navigate by at music festivals – started to fall away.

But although we had dark moments – how could you not? – we still, somehow, remained positive about the future. Even now, Zarah faced her predicament with stoicism, humour, charm and an indomitable spirit. 'Not letting cancer beat you' is such a tedious cliché, but she refused to. She was that stubborn.

Part of our coping mechanism was to fixate on two things: getting on to the BISCAY trial, and making it home in time to go on the next of our planned trips abroad: 10 days in the South of France, with a group of 10 of our closest friends, in mid-September.

And thanks to the nurses, the physios, the doctors, and Zarah's sheer bloody-mindedness, we made it on that holiday. It may have been the chemo, it may have been something shifting in Zarah's spine, it may have been in her mind, but after a few weeks, suddenly, over the course of a couple of days, Zarah's condition improved. To the delight of her physio, she walked up a flight of stairs unaided. Her back pain abated, as did the acute side effects of the chemo. Someone found some compression leggings – in a very fetching teal colour – which provided some partial respite from the lymphoedema. She was back in the game.

Earlier that summer, I'd signed up to run 10k to raise money for immunotherapy research. 'Race day' was on a Sunday in late August.

With the help of her friend Erin, some fentanyl, and a walking stick, Zarah made it out of hospital to wait for me at the finish line. As I came round the final bend, I saw her. Somehow, even though my legs were jelly, I managed a sprint finish, racing towards her, across the line. Surrounded by our friends and family, we had a massive, tearful, sweaty hug in the middle of Brockwell Park. Drained and dishevelled – but in nothing like the pain or anguish Zarah was in – I'd never cried for joy so hard as I did crossing that finish line.

I ended up raising £11,000, too.

Admission time: I've deliberately skipped a bit of the story. It goes better here, with the positivity of her imminent exit from hospital. But as a result, some of the facts in the previous section are slightly inaccurate: I referred to Zarah as a 37-year-old, and as my 'girlfriend'. But by the time she was admitted to Barts for that gruelling month, neither of those things was true.

On 15 August, shortly before that admission, Zarah turned 38. I took her out for a posh dinner, and while we waited for the bill, I asked her to marry me.

She said yes.

We were running very late. Well, technically, we were 'hobbling' late, or at least Zarah was. The train stretched out along the platform of Paris's Gare du Lyon, but only the distant carriages were leaving for Agen – and they were leaving in two minutes. I was grappling with two suitcases and a wheelchair that refused to go in the right direction. Zarah was limping along with a walking stick. The chair was my idea – 'just in case'. She steadfastly refused to use it. 'I'm not a fecking cripple, you know. I can still fecking walk!!'

'OK, fine, be a dick about it. Get on the train here, then! Walk down inside to our carriage. I'll wheel this down and meet you there.' I helped her on to the train, then sped up along the platform, wheelchair still determined to go one way, bags the other. Apart from Stu and Kate, whose two-year-old was delaying them even more than us (toddlers are more hassle than cancer patients, it seems), everyone else – Lindsey, David, David, Benjamin, Ben, and James and Annabell (who, by this point, was recovering well from her brain surgery) – was already on the train.

I just made it on board.

It had been a fight to get there: Zarah had finally been discharged from Barts two days previously. The nurses literally cheered for us. It was an emotional goodbye, but everyone knew we'd be back.

We'd got home with 48 hours to pack for France – no mean feat, given the complexity of Zarah's needs by then. She was still in a fair bit of discomfort and needed constant pain medication (although nothing like where she'd been a few weeks previously). The Barts team had drained the excess fluid from her right lymph node (more grist for the research mill) and it was far less throbby. Her appetite was returning. But her hair was now a few wispy blonde strands, covered with a red bandana. Her right leg was massive – now twice the weight of the left. She needed a cane to walk. She felt OK, but she looked…

…She looked like she had cancer.

I boarded the train at the appropriate carriage. All the gang was there, and Zarah was still hobbling along through the previous cars. Jon and Anna gave me a hand with the wheelchair.

Wait.

Jon? Anna?

Jon and Anna were Zarah's absolute best friends in the world.

They lived in Melbourne, Australia.

But they were here, on the train. In Paris.

Well played, guys.

Zarah finally arrived, took one look, and it was a beautiful scene. Pure happiness. Happy tears.

A cheese-baguette- and wine-fuelled train journey later, we picked up hire cars and drove to our destination – a beautiful old converted farmhouse in the French countryside. There was a swimming pool. We cooked incredible food every night. We convinced Jon and Anna's four-year-old son that Lindsey was an actual witch. One night, we all dressed up for a 'murder mystery' night – Zarah made a fabulous 'Misty Moon the fortune teller', and it turns out that I look pretty convincing as a clergyman (David did it).

One night, towards the end of the holiday, while everyone was making merry around the table, I snuck off to the end of the garden. I'm not superstitious and I don't believe in fate, but somehow – perhaps it was all the red wine – I felt compelled: I wanted to see a shooting star. I wanted to make a wish.

I waited and waited.

And waited.

I was getting chilly, but I carried on waiting – just standing there, gazing at the sky. It must have been 20 minutes or so.

There was no shooting star.

I rejoined everyone at the table, forcing a smile. The evening was winding down. A few hours later, we all went to bed.

A year later, on my own in North California, I finally saw a shooting star, and it broke my heart all over again.

By the time we got the train home, Zarah's back pain had returned with a vengeance. The morphine wasn't even touching the sides. The only thing that would relieve it was if I rubbed my hand in a circular motion round the small of her back. She leaned forwards and went to sleep with her face pressed against the seat in front. If I stopped rubbing, she'd wake with a start. It was a six-hour journey.

More worryingly, she was now only able to pee occasionally, even though her bladder felt constantly full. She had a minor but persistent nosebleed. And her leg was huge, and pitted when pressed. Six hours in a train seat did this no good at all. As wonderful as the holiday had been, I was relieved to be heading home. This all needed attention.

So for the third time, we got home, unpacked our holiday stuff, packed Zarah an overnight bag, and headed back to hospital. I'd called Tom – he'd booked Zarah a room in Barts Cancer Centre. This time, her bed was on the sister ward to where she'd been previously. I'll not be unkind about this adjacent ward, save to say Cinderella had sisters too.

Zarah was immediately sent for some scans – MRI and CT – and catheterised to help drain her bladder.

Tom came to see her the next day, to chat through where we were at. While we'd been away, he'd been consulting with all manner of specialists, looking at all Zarah's scans, blood test results, everything in the round. And, sitting next to Zarah's bed, leaning forwards intensely – glasses on, glasses off – he had lots to tell us.

First, the trial. AstraZeneca had finally processed Zarah's biopsy results. And as we'd suspected, in line with Charlie's findings back in February, her cancer didn't bear any of the mutations that matched the targeted drugs currently on offer, so she'd be getting immunotherapy on its own – OK, fine. The main issue now was that, for her to be formally accepted on to the trial and actually receive the drugs, she'd have to have blood test results that fell within very narrow parameters. Ninety per cent of the tests they'd run so far – liver function, kidney function, calcium levels, etc. – met these criteria. However, she was severely anaemic, and her blood clotting ability, as determined by her platelet levels, was way off.

In order to press the 'go' button on BISCAY, Tom's team just needed one set of 'perfect' results – across the board – to send to AZ. This was doable – she'd be given regular blood and platelet transfusions until everything was back within normal range, and we'd hope nothing else deteriorated in the process. This, I thought at the time, sounds a bit like cheating. But it also sounds quite easy. A few bags of blood and then boom – immunotherapy. OK. Cool. Let's do this.

Next, her bladder function. Although not directly part of the trial criteria, this needed sorting. The team suspected that the underlying cause was a large blood clot – or clots – in her bladder, so she'd need 'irrigating'. In practice, this somewhat agricultural term meant sticking a Y-shaped catheter through her urethra and into her bladder. One arm of the inverted 'Y' would be connected to a whopping great bag of saline drip, the other would go into a plastic bag attached to the lower rung of her hospital bed. They'd literally flush the clots out of her.

Finally, Tom wanted to talk about the cancer in her spine. 'I've been talking to some top radiologists about it. I was never completely convinced about the idea that it was cancer. And the good news is it's not.' Our jaws dropped. Instead, he said, the new MRI scans had revealed that it was most likely a long, thin blood clot, stretching the length of her spine. This, finally, explained why no one could give us an answer as to how many metastases there were. And why it suddenly cleared up. All the back-niggles Zarah had had in France had been just that. Niggles. Not cancer. Just a bad back.

No cancer in her spine. No paralysis. No wheelchair. That whole holiday, we'd had this unspoken future hanging over us needlessly. We were too shocked, too worn down to be angry. And why waste time on anger, when relief was a much better emotion?

But our relief was short-lived.

'There's bad news though. The latest CT scan tells me the cancer in your bladder is growing again, and it's spread to your liver.'

Fuck. OK.

Fuck.

Oh well. At least you definitely meet the trial criteria for progressive disease, we joked later, through clenched teeth.

It took a few days stuck in Barts for Zarah's bladder to be cleared out. The clots were huge, and would regularly block the catheter tube, necessitating its replacement. Those are easy words to type. It was horrible to have done. Zarah dealt with it, as always, with a grace and bravery that astounded us all.

A day into the irrigation, she developed another infection. More antibiotics. More delays. She'd need to stay.

Eventually, things ran clear ('Nice and yellow!' said one of the nurses, holding the bag up to the light) and the catheter was removed. Zarah's fluid intake was carefully recorded. No, let me rephrase – she carefully recorded her own fluid intake on a chart. When she'd wee, she'd have to measure it in a plastic jug. Then call a nurse, who, using a portable ultrasound machine, would measure how much urine was left in her bladder. Each time, there was still a substantial quantity of urine left. In the catheter would go, and we'd start again. This went on for several days. Eventually, it was decided that she'd probably need the catheter for the foreseeable future. Her infection had cleared up. She could go home. With a bag strapped to her leg for the catheter to empty into.

She'd had several bags of blood by this point, but her platelet levels, although much better, still weren't up to the magic level of 100. We'd have to come back for more in a day or so, but at least she could come home.

And so began a week in and out of Barts, as the team desperately, heroically pumped Zarah full of blood and platelets, and sent samples off for testing. Each time it inched nearer to the required values, but each time it was desperately short. By now we were both living in a state of high anxiety. Everything depended on this trial now. Everything.

As the team at Barts fought desperately to get Zarah on to the BISCAY trial, another depressing story was unfolding simultaneously. It's time to talk about lymphoedema.

I mentioned earlier I was angry about lymphoedema. Actually, I'm not angry, I'm filled with righteous burning rage, even today. The way our local NHS institutions currently manage cancer patients with lymphoedema, and its importance in the eyes of research funders, is a fucking scandal. It's a condition a huge proportion of cancer patients develop, and needs constant management. It's crippling, debilitating, and very difficult to manage. And yet, local lymphoedema services are often chronically underfunded, piecemeal, and disconnected from routine hospital and primary care. On top of this, research into lymphoedema treatment is, compared to research into other aspects of cancer, largely neglected. We'll get to how this affected Zarah in a minute, but first, I should probably explain what the bloody thing is. To paraphrase Matt Damon in the film *The Martian*: 'Let's physiology the shit out of it.'

If you did biology at school, you'll know about the circulatory system. It's pretty basic: your heart pumps blood through tubes around your body – arteries, veins, capillaries and all that. It's how oxygen gets from your lungs to your liver, how glucose gets from your digestive system to your muscles. Cut it and it bleeds. Simple, basic biology. Tubes carrying stuff, and a pump to pump it all around. You probably remember red blood cells, white blood cells, and maybe even systolic and diastolic pressures, atria and ventricles. Blood stuff. Heart stuff.

Just as important, but much less well understood by the general public, is the lymphatic system. It too is a network of tubes, carrying about 4 litres of a liquid called lymph around the body from where it's made to where it's needed. Just like the circulatory system, it has a number of disparate functions – in this case, it's a waste disposal system, it maintains the fluid balance in your tissues, and acts as a conduit for important components of your immune system.

But unlike the circulatory system, it doesn't have a pump. Instead, it relies on your movement – walking around, waving your arms, dancing like a loon at a music festival – to slowly move the lymph around.

You've probably also heard of your 'lymph nodes' (at the very least, if you've been paying attention to this book you will have). They're the bits of you that get swollen when you get an infection and are often, colloquially, called 'glands' (a bit of a misnomer, as there are other types of gland, like your thyroid, that have nothing to do with the lymph system, but I digress). Even though you're probably only familiar with the ones in your throat and groin, the human body contains hundreds of them (between 500 and 700, depending on the individual). They're everywhere.

These hundreds of lymph nodes do a whole bunch of different things (such as nurturing certain types of immune cell), but for this bit of the story we need to focus on one very important function – they're your tissues' filters. Excess water in any of your body tissues is carried by the lymph vessels to the nodes, then to a duct in your thorax, where it enters your blood, then carried away to the kidneys, where it's extracted and flows into your bladder. Then, if you're lucky, you wee it out.

So, to recap: the lymph system is basically a drain, and its nodes are its filters. And it turns out cancer cells *love* them. In most types of cancer, the first sign it's spreading is when rogue cancer cells take up residence in nearby lymph nodes and start multiplying, clogging them up. In some cancer types, these clogged nodes can be removed with surgery – but that means blocking one of the exit points from the drain. So, clogged or missing, this can cause the system to back up. Lymphoedema is, ultimately, a condition caused by the physiological equivalent of a blocked filter in your dishwasher.

If you've ever had a blocked dishwasher, you know what happens. Everything fills up with waste water. Everything gets sodden. Everything gets ruined. And so it is with lymphoedema.

This is a necessarily simplified description, but you get the picture. In people with breast cancer, the surgical removal of lymph nodes from the armpit – either to diagnose or treat the disease – can mean they get lymphoedema in their arm. When Annabell had the lymph nodes removed from her groin to try to halt the spread of her melanoma, she developed lymphoedema in her leg. Ever since, she's needed to wear a compression stocking to keep it under control.

In Zarah's case, clogged, cancer-filled lymph nodes in her groin and abdomen meant the fluid in her legs – fluid that collects there in each and every one of us, every day – couldn't drain. Every glass of water she drank, every meal she ate, put more fluid into her body – and only a fraction of it would come out the other end. Add the fact that she couldn't pee properly due to the progressing tumour in her bladder, and the result was a particularly nasty, progressive condition. On its own, cancer aside, it's enough to kill you – and in fact, it was most likely the build-up of fluid that played a key role at the end.

So, you'd have thought that such a nasty, progressive, debilitating – yet common – condition in cancer patients would attract the attention of senior specialists, have entire wards dedicated to it, not to mention research programmes, trials, international consortia. Maybe Joe Biden would promise to stick it on the fucking moon. Right?

Wrong. What there was on offer to cancer patients with lymphoedema in Tower Hamlets, Hackney and Newham in 2016 was, when all is said and done, a lone, highly trained but desperately overstretched young woman with a Travelcard, who carried a large backpack in which was to be found a plastic stress ball and some bandages.

Don't get me wrong, Anna was brilliant. She knew her stuff. She really cared. She and Zarah really got on. She did absolutely everything she could. But she was hampered by two things.

First, treatment for lymphoedema is still in the Dark Ages compared with most other aspects of cancer. There are no specific drugs, unless you count diuretics (which just make you pee more – not much use if the problem is literally upstream). There's no surgery that can replumb the blocked drains (at least, not yet). So the main option for Zarah – as for most people with lymphoedema – was something called 'lymphatic drainage massage', together with compression garments.

Lymphatic drainage massage, unlike other forms of massage, is deeply unsexy. It involves placing a squishy stress ball – the sort handed out at conferences – next to a partially blocked node in, say, the groin, and pressing into it, to squeeze the fluid past the blockage into the blood. Then, using the edge of your hand, you physically scoop the fluid up the leg towards the now empty node. It's really weird to do. I got quite good at it. In Zarah's case, it would take me about half an hour to 'do' each leg, and provided about an hour's relief before everything swelled up again. It was basically Sisyphean, although I'm not sure Zarah would have liked me comparing her legs to boulders. And this was because the arrival of the second component of lymphoedema treatment – compression garments – was unfortunately delayed.

Compression garments for lymphoedema of the legs are basically very, very tight leggings. The really good ones are made to measure (you can get them in all sorts of crazy patterns – Zarah was quite excited) and you need to wear them all the time (although you can take them off for the drainage massage, and for washing, etc.). You can probably guess how they work, but in case not: they continually squeeze the fluid out of the given limb, like a constant drainage massage. In August, during her long stint on Ward 5A, Zarah had been given a pair of generic compression stockings. But as things progressed, they became unusable – partly because they just moved the fluid from her calves up to her thighs, but also because, as Zarah's legs got bigger, they were an absolute nightmare to get on.

The other thing hampering Anna's ability to treat Zarah's lymphoedema was purely bureaucratic, and perhaps the thing that enrages me most. Here come some acronyms. Anna worked for a non-profit called Accelerate CIC, which was commissioned (NHS-speak for being paid for) by the local Clinical Commissioning Group, or CCG – a conglomerate of local GPs in Tower Hamlets responsible for managing a big chunk of the NHS budget. This difference in paymasters and geography meant Anna was, frustratingly, not allowed to see Zarah while she lay in her bed in Barts, for reasons that were never made clear to us. Let me reiterate that: Anna was *contractually forbidden* from seeing Zarah while she was an inpatient at Barts. But Barts itself has no lymphoedema services, as these are all managed 'in the community' by people like Anna. So we had the FUCKING RIDICULOUS situation where Zarah was lying in a hospital bed, slowly swelling up, but unable to be measured for compression garments that would help her until she was discharged… but one of the reasons she couldn't be discharged was that her mobility was impaired by her lymphoedema.

Paging Kafka. We've got a good one for you.

The upshot of it was this: despite Zarah's lymphoedema being a serious clinical issue from about early August, she didn't see a specialist – Anna – until late September, just after we got back from France. Add to that the several-week turnaround time for the compression garments to be manufactured in Germany and posted to London, and you get to mid-October. And by the time the stockings finally arrived, things were progressing rapidly, and Zarah was now too big to wear them safely. To do so would have been downright dangerous – it could have pushed all the water on to her abdomen and into her lungs.

You can see why I'm fucking angry.

Oh, wait, another thing. When Zarah was discharged from Barts, ready to go to the South of France, she was given a now familiar green-and-white Macmillan booklet, this time entitled 'Understanding Lymphoedema'.

OK, we should have read it. We had a lot going on. It got ignored.

I finally got round to flicking through it when we were back in London, after 10 days sitting in the sun, eating evening meals al fresco, and wandering around a brambly garden.

Buried towards the back of the booklet, three facts leaped out at me (I paraphrase Macmillan's normally oh-so-polite tone):

- DON'T GET SUNBURNT
- DON'T GET MOSQUITO BITES
- DON'T LET YOUR SKIN GET DAMAGED

Any of these things, the booklet said, can trigger something truly horrible called lymphorroea – a non-healing gash that continually oozes lymph, and is a huge infection risk.

You'd have thought someone might have mentioned this to Zarah before we went to the SOUTH OF FUCKING FRANCE.

Le sigh.

So that's my lymphoedema rage out the way. Sorry about that.

To add to the complex picture, we need to add the other community services Zarah now needed to avail herself of. Zarah's GP was involved in prescribing various non-essential but useful lotions and potions (laxatives, nappy-rash cream, moisturisers), keeping track of Zarah's overall mental well-being, and, well, doing GP stuff. St Joseph's were in charge of Zarah's painkillers. Anna was leading on the lymphoedema management. And occasionally we'd need the local district nurses – out-of-hours medical professionals who would come to the flat and change dressings and catheters (since her last stay in Barts, Zarah now had a permanent catheter – at least it saved her a trip up the stairs for a pee).

The trouble was, these four distinct bits of the NHS were, well, just that. Distinct. The district nurses were paid for by the local council. The GP was part of the local CCG. St Joseph's is an independent charity, contracted by local NHS Trusts (i.e. hospitals). Anna's company, Accelerate-CIC, was contracted by the GP-led CCG. It was a mess, and nothing felt joined up. So Zarah took matters into her own hands and called what could be effectively described as a *Loya Jirga* – a tribal gathering of disparate community healthcare professionals. She literally diary-managed the lot of them by phone until they could agree a date to all visit our flat. Together. At the same time.

Zarah was reclined on our sofa. Next to her was our lead palliative care nurse from St Joseph's. Fiona, our wonderful GP, was sitting on the pouffe. Standing in the corner was one of the district nurses – a terse lady, whose name I forget. Anna was crouched on the floor next to Zarah with her ever-present backpack. I pulled over a chair from the dining table. The room was buzzing – ideas bounced off each other, mobile numbers were swapped. Of particular note, Fiona and Anna had a long conversation about whether to prescribe Zarah diuretics. We pointed out that various things were off limits because of the trial criteria. Fiona said she'd speak to Tom. Finally, it felt like we were getting integrated care. Zarah had, as she always did, brought people together to make the world better – this time, admittedly, for herself, but still.

And then, catheter-gate happened.

Zarah had just come home from Barts, infection-free, pain much better controlled, but carrying a catheter bag. This was even less dignified than the nephrostomy – a thick plastic tube protruding from her knickers carrying urine to a bag on her leg. It chafed. You've never known love till you've moisturised your fiancée's catheter sores – trust me.

We were constantly paranoid that the catheter would block. I continually checked the volume of urine in it, to make sure things were flowing as they should. We'd even worked out how to flush the tube ourselves. I won't go into the details – they're even less romantic than the previous paragraph. But there is no sense of shared achievement in a relationship like successfully unblocking your fiancée's bladder and avoiding a trip to A&E.

Sadly, just two days back from Barts, and the catheter blocked – properly this time, beyond my self-taught syringe skills. And so began the episode that was one of the most harrowing, upsetting and devastating of the entire story – not only for Zarah, but for me too. Zarah said to a friend later that it was when she saw my optimism and resolve finally break. I just remember the look on her face, and the noise she made, while He Was Doing It.

It was about 10 p.m. We'd had a lovely chilled evening in front of the telly. I'd cooked us something nice, but I forget what. Then, suddenly, Zarah felt like she was swelling up. She was distressed. I checked – nothing was coming out of her catheter. I tried unblocking it with a syringe, but no joy. We called the district nurse. As per usual, a brusque woman with a terrible bedside manner showed up a few hours later, with another in tow – we never ascertained whether she too was a nurse, or just her friend. It was gone midnight. Zarah lay on the sofa, skirt hitched up, naked from the waist down, as the nurse removed the catheter, stuck a new one in and wiggled it around a bit to try to get things flowing. Nothing. She tried flushing it with saline. Nothing. She removed the new catheter and tried again with a second one (the discarded catheter was dropped into a plastic bag by the sofa).

Still nothing. Try again. Flush. No. And again.

Eventually: 'I cannot make it work. You must go to A&E. I call you an ambulance.'

The paramedics arrived after 15 awkward minutes, and the nurse briefed them on Zarah's situation, before departing swiftly, leaving discarded catheters, syringes, surgical gloves, etc. in a plastic bag next to the sofa.

While I packed another overnight bag, the paramedics (who were lovely) strapped Zarah into a stretcher and carried her to the lift. I followed them down. The blue lights were flashing – neighbours peered over the balcony.

In The London's A&E we had a long wait for a cubicle, but eventually were seen by a mildly charmless young Australian nurse, who had another crack at catheterising and flushing Zarah's bladder with a series of ever-wider tubes. Still no joy. Zarah was starting to feel really swollen now. And yet she did not complain once.

We were moved to another room, and He arrived. The Urologist.

He was a young (I guessed) Eastern European or Russian doctor. I hadn't thought it possible to have a worse bedside manner than either of the previous two. But He did.

He barely said a word, He just set about Zarah's nether regions, trying to catheterise and flush, just as everyone else had.

He'd brought with him a portable ultrasound machine, to try to assess how much liquid was in her bladder, but He couldn't get it to work – it was a different model, apparently, to the one He was used to.

'I try to break clot,' He informed us, before drawing out a terrifying-looking 2-foot-long metal wire from a trolley next to him.

He stuck this down the catheter tube into Zarah's bladder and repeatedly jabbed hard and wiggled it around. I held her hand while He thrusted.

Each time, she'd recoil. Each time, she'd bite back a scream. Jab, wiggle, jab, wiggle. I held her hand. He kept jabbing. She kept recoiling.

We looked into each other's eyes as He thrusted the wire into her bladder, and part of me died.

'Hmm, still not working. Maybe she needs a scan.'

'What? Haven't you looked at the CT she had last week?' I implored.

'She has scan? OK, I go find.'

We sat in silence. There was nothing to say.

He came back.

'OK, is not blood clot. Blockage is probably the cancer. You need to go to urology.'

The Urologist had spent several minutes brutalising Zarah's tumour with a metal wire for no reason. There was no 'blockage'. There was just no space left in her bladder.

We got up to a urology bed at 5 a.m. We were both tearful and traumatised. Zarah went straight to sleep. I took one of the spare pillows from her bed and – utterly broken – curled up on the cold, hard floor of her room and did likewise.

The next few weeks were a blur. I've pieced together the events from a range of sources – my Google calendar, appointment letters from various bits of the NHS, WhatsApp messages, Facebook posts, my own shattered memory. This is what happened next.

Zarah came home from the Royal London's urology ward and we bunkered down in our flat. She now had a permanent catheter, out of which came a constant trickle of bloody urine. We had two challenges ahead of us: getting her fit for the BISCAY trial, and managing her bladder issues. The former was to involve a few more blood and platelet transfusions, and a lot of finger-crossing. For the latter, Zarah was referred to the urology outpatient clinic, where she'd be taught to self-catheterise, and monitored regularly. All we wanted to do was curl up and hide from the world, but we were juggling appointments between two hospitals – Barts for the transfusions, plus a last-minute heart scan to check she had no underlying issues; The London for the urology stuff. We waited for the lymphoedema stockings to arrive, which would hopefully bring some relief and mobility.

Zarah was now permanently drowsy from the painkillers, and would occasionally drift off mid-sentence. I'd have to help her with her text messages and emails, as her coordination was so scrambled. Getting out and about meant a wheelchair – the one we'd taken to France but not used. Thanks to the lymphoedema and her slothful bladder, and because her blood's capacity to transport water was being eroded by her cancer,* fluid was starting to accumulate in her lungs, so unless she slept

---

*Water is carried in the blood by a protein called albumin. Cancers tend to consume this as fuel, so its levels can drop in advanced disease – something that worsens as people get very sick and lose their appetite, meaning they can't replace the lost albumin. A horrible, vicious, lethal circle.

in a semi-sitting position, propped up by several pillows, her breathing would become difficult.

Psychologically, it was a bizarre, surreal place to be. Even more so than before, our coping mechanism was to look ahead to the next appointment and not much beyond that. Upon learning we'd got engaged, a few people asked us if we'd set a date. It was a question I just couldn't process. It had no meaning. Nothing other than the trial mattered now.

And yet, somehow, we stayed optimistic. We'd get through this. We would. All this was temporary. Normal service would be resumed. There was light at the end of the tunnel, and its name was immunotherapy. This was a fact I believed with a certainty that, in retrospect, seems almost evangelical. Hope is a powerful thing. Too powerful? Maybe, but what have you got without it?

One memory from the urology appointment sticks out. The large, spacious upper-floor waiting room, which has a gorgeous view across London. It was a beautiful, sunny day. The clouds had cleared. You could see for miles. It felt like a sign. We played 'spot the landmark' while we waited. We were in good spirits, as usual.

The appointment itself involved both Zarah and I learning how to locate the entrance to her urethra, in her now-swollen vulva, and insert a thin temporary catheter bag. She'd have to do this every time she needed a pee, and it'd mean she could get rid of the permanent bag. Zarah managed it first time, I managed it second time. Success. We could do anything. This was just one more surreal event in our now surreal existence. We took it, as with everything else, in our stride.

My mum came to visit us in the flat. It was the first time she'd seen Zarah since before our trip to France, and she was visibly shocked at her appearance. Thanks to her lack of appetite, her top half was wasting away; her lower half was massive. So gradual had been the change, I hadn't noticed. I remember writing Mum's reaction off as her usual tendency towards the melodramatic.

On Wednesday 11 October, we had a phone call from the research nurse at Barts, giving us the good news. The results of the latest blood test were back: Zarah's platelet levels had passed 100. AstraZeneca had formally accepted her on to the BISCAY trial. Could we come in tomorrow to have the first dose?

I sent the news to our friends and family, accompanied by a photo: two glasses of champagne, clinking together. You could see Zarah's engagement ring sparkling on her slender finger: a gorgeous vintage jade and diamond affair that had been my grandmother's – a gift from my mum, who'd been saving it for me. It looked amazing on her, complementing her eyes perfectly. She adored it. What you couldn't see in the photo was the clear plastic spacers on the underside of the ring, preventing it from falling off, so much weight had she lost.

We still hoped to make it to Spain for Alex's birthday – a bit later than planned, but that's cancer for you. I called easyJet and rearranged our flights.

Having immunotherapy turned out to be exactly as unexceptional as having chemotherapy – a colourless bag of liquid administered via an IV drip into Zarah's PICC line. Pramit turned up to get some more blood and urine samples for his and Sophia's research. He'd later tell me that, seeing Zarah that day, he knew. But our optimism was palpable. He said nothing, and I'm forever glad that he, and everyone else, held their tongue.

Two days after Zarah had immunotherapy, on a Friday night, I had a night off from my job of constant carer, and went with Lindsey to see my friend Kieran's sold-out show at the Brixton Academy – an all-nighter of DJ sets, with Kieran headlining. I needed it. Zarah knew I needed it. He'd got us access-all-areas VIP passes. I've known him since we were both five years old. His family were all there, and they showered me with love and affection. Lindsey and I got smashed. I remember a small thought flashing through my head: this is what going out without Zarah's going to be like – get used to it. I extinguished it as soon as it appeared.

I got home in the small hours. Zarah was still awake – both of our sleep patterns were all over the place. I asked her how she was. 'It's blocked again,' she said. We agreed to give it a few hours – time for me to get some sleep – then try again when I woke up. If we couldn't get it sorted, we'd call it in. I kissed her goodnight and curled up asleep in the crook of her emaciated arm.

The alarm went off several hours later. Zarah woke me with a kiss. 'I still can't pee.'

I texted Tom Powles for advice then packed a hospital bag, for what would turn out to be the last time.

VIII: Dominance

The monster has regenerated

Its vast mass fills the bladder once more, and – thanks to its regrown network of capillaries – is constantly releasing its lethal progeny into the bloodstream, to travel far and wide. These cells – great, great, and greater grandchildren of the long-deceased mother cell – all carry her hallmark complement of genetic faults, along with scores more. New superpowers, awakened as it accelerated chaotically back in the aftermath of its epic battle for survival.

One fault, recently accrued, in different ways in different lineages of cells – parallell evolution in action – has further supercharged the monster's growth rate. Another activates previously suppressed circuitry, coating the cells in immune-suppressing markers.

The inflamed, bleeding mass grows unhindered. Billions of cells, growing exponentially, spreading, penetrating, shedding.

In vain, the cells of the immune system attack what they can, blind to the vast majority of the monster's mass. They are hopelessly outnumbered, outgunned, outmanoeuvred, and exhausted.

The monster's dominance is complete. Short of a miracle, its growth is now unstoppable.

It's 4 p.m. on a rainy October afternoon. I'm in an isolated little cabin in the Surrey Hills staring at a blank laptop screen. I've come here to write. It's been a week, and I've got loads done. But today, the cabin is spotless – I've been procrastinating all afternoon, because this is going to be the hardest bit of this book to write. But write it I must – this story needs telling. If you're going to understand cancer properly, you need to know how it ends. Here we go… deep breath, this is the saddest bit.

Tom called me back quickly, even though it was a Saturday. He desperately wanted Zarah to go to Barts – he could easily arrange her a bed in the ward there, and the team were fully up to speed with her case and predicament. But Barts has no urology department, and her issues were primarily urological. We'd have to go to The London again – our least favourite of the four hospitals Zarah'd been to. Even though

Barts and The London are part of the same NHS Trust, Tom has no jurisdiction over admissions at the latter, so we'd have to go via A&E.

The wait for a bed wasn't too long. Zarah was transferred up to the ward later on Saturday afternoon. A CT scan was ordered and carried out. I stayed with her until early evening, until she drifted off to sleep – then went home to do likewise.

I headed back in on Sunday lunchtime. It was a beautiful day. Tom rang to discuss the scan results, and I left Zarah's ward to take the call in the family waiting room, which was, thankfully, empty.

'I don't think this is going to work,' he said.

'What, the immunotherapy? I thought it works in 20 per cent of patients, has something changed?' I stared out the window at the view, unable to process the words I was hearing.

'No, I just mean, I think things are progressing quite quickly now.'

Tom explained how, in patients in whom they worked, these drugs often took a while to have an effect, as the immune system could take several weeks to get up to speed.

'But in others it works quite quickly, doesn't it?' Yes, said Tom. 'So there's still hope.'

'Yes, but we're in a very tricky situation now, Henry.'

My ears were hearing, but my brain wasn't understanding. If there was still hope, there was still hope. End of.

The urology team had managed to get Zarah's bladder draining, and it was decided that she'd now be better off in Barts. An ambulance was called, and she was wheeled down and out into it. We cracked jokes with the paramedics – I can't remember about what, but I remember laughing a lot. Still. Even then.

In Barts, the oncology team explained what the scan had shown. Many more growths in Zarah's liver. More extensive growth throughout her pelvis. More lymph nodes. The penny had been tossed, was spinning – heads or tails, live or die – but, for me at least, still hadn't dropped.

The next morning I overslept. I think by this point I was beyond exhausted, ready to crash, but still going. As long as she needed me, I'd keep going. But I think that morning was the first morning I failed her. I woke to the phone ringing. It was Zarah. 'Can you come in? Tom's here and wants to talk. He'll be coming round in about half an hour. Hurry.'

I hurried. But not enough. By the time I got there, he'd left – I passed him in the corridor, but he was talking earnestly to another senior oncologist and he didn't see me. I didn't want to interrupt.

I got to Zarah's bed, and she was sitting up, alert and awake. She greeted me cheerfully, but something had changed. It looked a bit like she'd been crying.

'I had an awful night's sleep – it's so noisy in here.'

I told her I'd seen Tom in the corridor. 'Go and grab him!' she urged. I refused – he was busy, and I wanted to be with her. She looked like she needed me.

Frustrated, Zarah calmly told me the new plan: it was far too hectic in Barts, so they'd arranged to transfer her to a bed at the more peaceful St Joseph's. There was no clinical reason for her to be taking up an oncology bed – at St Joe's they could keep her stable and give the drugs a chance to work.

She'd be transferred later that day.

It was only later – much later – that I realised what Tom had actually told Zarah. It was – is – the single most painful recollection I have of her whole illness. I'd been there with her at every step of the way, for every new twist and turn cancer threw at us. The diagnosis. The mid-treatment and final treatment scans. Deciding which trial to go on. Getting on the trial.

But for the one piece of news that really mattered, I was at home, asleep, and she had to hear it on her own. I try not to, but I beat myself up about this every day.

When she heard she was going to die, she was on her own. Team Twat, separated for the crucial play.

———

By this point, in addition to being Zarah's chief carer, drug administrator, catheteriser, jargon-translator and pillow-fluffer, I was also her diary manager. So many people wanted to visit her, and I was responsible for telling them where and when. I put the word out she was going to be in St Joseph's Hospice.

I think everyone twigged what was going on. The word 'hospice' will do that. But I still hadn't. The penny continued to spin.

OK, I had an inkling. Of course I did. I phoned Zarah's sister and told her the news. She marshalled the rest of her family – including the frail and elderly Sean – on to a Ryanair flight from Cork. My mum, who was on holiday in Italy, got the next flight back. My dad flew in from Marrakech, where he'd been at a conference. Likewise, Lindsey – abroad with work, but due to meet us in Spain – flew back too.

Slowly, the waiting room opposite Zarah's room at St Joseph's filled up with a gang of beautiful people – all our family, our best friends – all ashen-faced, but being brave. There was so much love in that room – along with several tons of food sent over from Zarah's colleagues at M&S. It was like the oddest party in the world.

But I knew we didn't need to be brave. The drugs would work. I just knew.

The nurses made me up a bed in Zarah's room. They upped her painkillers, and she drifted out of consciousness more regularly.

We took it in shifts. My mum was offered a bed in the guest bedroom up the corridor. Amber, Michael, Florence and Sean were staying nearby and were there most of the time, as was my dad. A few of us would occasionally go off to the pub for a breather, just a text message away if anything should change. And for three days, nothing did.

On the second day, however, I had an extraordinary, surreal conversation with Dr Maggie. She wanted to let me know they wanted to put a 'Do not resuscitate' mark in Zarah's notes. This meant, should anything change, they wouldn't call an ambulance to take her to A&E.

I just couldn't understand. She'd just, last week, been pumped full of immunotherapy – we needed to give those drugs every hour, every second, to work. If that meant strapping her up to a ventilator and a machine that goes bing down in A&E, then we had to do that. Why give up? We'd come so far. We'd fought so hard. Maggie explained the distress this could cause, set against the chances of success. Alien words like 'futile' rang through my ears – but again, my brain couldn't quite grasp the situation. It wasn't my decision. It was Maggie's. Reluctantly, I agreed.

But I still hoped. Round and round span the penny, hanging in mid-air. Heads or tails. Life or death.

Later that day, we arranged for Zarah's bed to be wheeled down to the hospice's garden, a host of us in tow. I remembered how Zarah had spoken fondly about this place – how she'd sit there after her counselling sessions, and think, and come to terms with what was happening. Despite the fact that she was now pretty much permanently zonked out on the painkillers, unable to hold a conversation, barely able to focus, we figured that a bit of fresh air would do her the power of good. Some friends had brought some cans of gin and tonic to help pass the time in the waiting room – there were two left. We took them with us. I gave one to Florence, and took the other for Zarah and I to share.

We spent half an hour in the garden, Zarah almost completely unconscious, unaware what was going on, oblivious to the tranquil calm of the garden around us. It was getting cold, and the sun had set. Florence finished her can – I'd drunk half of mine. 'I don't think she'll want it,' said Florence.

Quick as a flash, an arm extended from the bed, grasping the can from my hand.

'Yes, I fucking will,' said Zarah.

———

That night, they wheeled in an extra bed, and set it level with Zarah's. We spent the night together, my arms wrapped around her now emaciated frame, her breathing ever more ragged, as the fluid slowly filled up her body. To try to keep my mind engaged with something – anything – I listened to *Test Match Special* on headphones throughout the night. England vs Bangladesh. Stokes took four wickets. I struggled to care.

The following day came and went. But something had changed in Zarah's breathing. It was a bit more rattly.

'I don't think it'll be much longer now,' one of the nurses told me.

The penny, suspended in mid-air, finally, at long last, landed.

———

It was late – gone midnight. Most of the gang had left the hospice, but Amber and Michael were still there, keeping watch.

Lindsey, James and a few others had come back with me to the flat, to keep me company with a bottle of Irish whiskey. At 2 a.m., my phone rang. It was one of the nurses. We should come back.

Everyone waited outside, across the corridor in the family room. I went in alone, me and Zarah, Team Twat, together till the end. I pressed my forehead against hers, willing the T-cells in her body to multiply, to start killing the cancer cells ravaging her body. I could practically visualise them. Even then, at the end, there was still a flame of hope flickering in a tiny corner of my mind. Come on, Zarah, I know you're usually late, but this is getting ridiculous.

I brought up the lyrics to Sufjan Stevens' 'Chicago' on my phone, its glow illuminating our faces in the darkness. And, as her breathing became more and more ragged, I sang her our song, one last time.

All things go. All things go.

And then, just like that, she went.

6

Waves a hundred feet tall

G RIEF IS A TAPESTRY of the cruellest paradoxes and ironies – a fundamentally, universally, essentially human experience for which nothing can prepare you. It's raw, soul-wrenching, devastating, isolating, crushing, agonising – a cascading loneliness that rips apart your being and forces you to remake it. I'm almost of a mind not to even try to capture it with the written word: as I was to discover, others have written more profoundly, more beautifully, of grief and loss than I can possibly hope to do. For example, CS Lewis, in *A Grief Observed* – a book pressed almost wordlessly into my hands by a close friend at Zarah's memorial – pretty much nails it:

> *'One flesh. Or, if you prefer, one ship. The starboard engine has gone. I, the port engine, must chug along somehow till we make harbour. Or rather, till the journey ends. How can I assume a harbour? A lee shore, more likely, a black night, a deafening gale, breakers ahead – and any lights shown from the land probably being waved by wreckers.'*

The shipwreck metaphor feels apt, although I have barely been sailing in my life. Perhaps the most perfect summary I stumbled across, in those first, lonely, lost few months, one from which I drew immense comfort, I found – bizarrely enough – on the online forum Reddit, posted by a user called GSnow:

> *'You'll find [grief] comes in waves. When the ship is first wrecked, you're drowning, with wreckage all around you. Everything floating around you reminds you of the beauty and the magnificence of the ship that was, and is no more. And all you can do is float. You find some piece of the wreckage and you hang on for a while. Maybe*

it's some physical thing. Maybe it's a happy memory or a photograph. Maybe it's a person who is also floating. For a while, all you can do is float. Stay alive.

'In the beginning, the waves are 100 feet tall and crash over you without mercy. They come 10 seconds apart and don't even give you time to catch your breath. All you can do is hang on and float. After a while, maybe weeks, maybe months, you'll find the waves are still 100 feet tall, but they come further apart. When they come, they still crash all over you and wipe you out. But in between, you can breathe, you can function. You never know what's going to trigger the grief. It might be a song, a picture, a street intersection, the smell of a cup of coffee. It can be just about anything... and the wave comes crashing. But in between waves, there is life.

'Somewhere down the line, and it's different for everybody, you find that the waves are only 80 feet tall. Or 50 feet tall. And while they still come, they come further apart. You can see them coming. An anniversary, a birthday, or Christmas, or landing at O'Hare. You can see it coming, for the most part, and prepare yourself. And when it washes over you, you know that somehow you will, again, come out the other side. Soaking wet, sputtering, still hanging on to some tiny piece of the wreckage, but you'll come out. Take it from an old guy. The waves never stop coming, and somehow you don't really want them to. But you learn that you'll survive them. And other waves will come. And you'll survive them too. If you're lucky, you'll have lots of scars from lots of loves. And lots of shipwrecks.'

Zarah had just died of cancer. The phrase roiled around my consciousness, mantra-like, as the metaphorical waves battered into my being. My girlfriend – my fiancée – had just died of cancer. Our team was shattered. I had no idea what was supposed to happen next. I didn't want to know. I just wanted to curl up into a tiny ball of tense, shrieking agony and collapse in on myself like a sad, lonely star imploding under its own gravity.

But I couldn't. Not yet. We had practical matters to attend to.

It turns out that one of the most unbearable aspects of the deep-seated social ritual we perform when someone dies is the bureaucracy that flows in its wake: death certificates, funerals, crematoriums, undertakers, catering, guest lists and the rest. Just when you want to shut down and weep, to hide, to mourn, to curl up and scream... you have to navigate the most extraordinary, unknown, unknowable administrative duties. It feels like a bug, not a feature, although I'm sure there's some rationale that it 'keeps you busy'.

Nevertheless, we were determined to make sure Zarah went out with a glorious, celebratory bang.

Of course – of *course* – there had to be a massive, fuck-off party. It's What She Would Have Wanted. But she would also have wanted a Quaker ceremony. And she'd wanted to be cremated. And there were literally hundreds of people who wanted to pay their respects, to mourn her loss, to share their memories. How on earth to square this circle? Particularly since, given how swiftly and brutally the previous few weeks had unfolded, through an opiate-induced cloud of hope and shock, Zarah hadn't had time to leave detailed instructions.

The answer was simple: do all of it. It's what she would have wanted. It's what I wanted. And, also, it was Something To Do. Feature, not bug, after all.

In retrospect, I just do not know how we pulled it off. There were several parallel WhatsApp groups. Everyone mucked in – of course they did – and in the end we did something pretty special, that will live on in the memories of everyone who was there, almost as vividly as does the memory of the incredible, irreplaceable woman whose life and loss we felt so beholden to honour.

First, the cremation. Zarah's sister, Amber, and her husband, Michael, heroically, stoically took on the task of sorting out all the paperwork and form-filling. Zarah's mum, Lindsey and I met prospective funeral directors. It was to be a relatively small, intimate service, for close friends and family. Potential slots at the City of London Crematorium were held. Poems were sourced. Spreadsheets were shared. Names were collated. Flights were booked. A coffin was chosen. Flowers were ordered. A website was constructed. Music was selected.

Then the memorial. With Florence's help, we found the largest Quaker Meeting House in East London – by happy coincidence, ten minutes' walk from the crematorium. I read up on the norms and etiquettes of Quaker funerals: as with Sunday worship, the idea is Quakerly simple – an hour's silent reflection, during which time people may share reflections, but no singing; no prayer. More flowers ordered. More names collated – a wider list than for the cremation. We wanted everyone to have a chance to remember.

Next, the party. Just to be difficult, I had decided that She Would Have Wanted live music. She would have wanted something extraordinary, glamorous and over the top. And inside me, I knew for certain: I had to sing 'Chicago' for her, one last time. I reached out – yes, for once that term is appropriate: I was grasping, lost, and desperate – to my old band, and to a small number of close musical friends of ours, including Annabell's boyfriend, James. We struggled to find a venue – we wanted something that could hold a few hundred, that had a late licence, and a stage. And a bar. Of course, a bar. After a few attempts, we found the perfect spot: Bethnal Green Working Men's Club, just round the corner from our flat. Shabby. Kitsch. Camp. A disco ball. A stage bearing a huge illuminated heart. So Zarah. It's What She Would Have Wanted.

Plan made, venues identified, the final step was to find a mutually acceptable date for all three. Happily, the stars aligned: just over two weeks after her death, on a Friday, all three places were free. We pressed the metaphorical 'go' button – and something extraordinary came to pass.

Perhaps fuelled by a collective, grief-induced mania, perhaps by love, everything, everybody, miraculously, ran like clockwork. Scores of our friends mucked in. A huge decorating crew was assembled. Photos were collated. A booklet was produced and printed. Catering was booked. Rehearsals were scheduled. A sound system was donated, and its donors, two dear friends of Lindsey's (and, by extension, mine and Zarah's), agreed to manage the sound on the night. Limos and a hearse were booked. Invitations were sent. Zarah's old Dutchie bike, decrepit and rusty, was polished up and bedecked with fairy lights and flowers. Two weeks came and went. The band even squeezed in two whole rehearsals. Everything was in place.

During the wait, a political bombshell was lobbed into our already shell-shocked lives: Trump, not Hillary. It felt like Zarah had abandoned us to party in the heavens with Bowie and Prince, leaving us on Earth to make our own fun amid unspeakable hellfire and division. (In truth, the 24-hour transatlantic news cycle was a welcome distraction from my own tortures.)

And, despite these darkening clouds, the day itself – although I have very little memory of it, being as I was barely held together with Sellotape, string and love – was perfection. The cremation was heart-wrenchingly, mournfully beautiful: after a beautiful eulogy from

Amber, and a poem from Lindsey, Zarah's coffin disappeared behind the curtain to the inappropriately appropriate 'Get Lucky' by Daft Punk, drawing irreverent, knowing giggles from half our friends. We could almost hear her cackle. Inside the coffin, she was dressed in the purple dress with the frilly red underskirt, clutching an empty can of M&S gin and tonic.

The Quaker ceremony was an outpouring of wonderful, sad, devastating, beautiful memories – from her best friends, from the homeless borrowers from the Quaker Mobile Library, from Sophia, from my mother, from so many more. I wanted to share, but I found myself pinned to my seat with grief, Mum holding my hand comfortingly. I have no idea what I would have said, although I'd mulled over something about Zarah's memory meaning that, with the advent of Brexit and now Trump, we should sow love not hate. But it felt too trite. Too political. I wasn't sure it's what she would have wanted.

Florence's mobile went off loudly in the middle of the silent reflection. Of course it did.

And the party: a glorious, sparkling, drunken outpouring of love and grief; a collective willing of her spirit into us all to dance, drink, smile, laugh, strut, just as she would have. Her bike, in the corner, twinkling and unridden. Erin and the rest of Zarah's marvellous team heroically orchestrated the delivery of a cornucopia of catering, donated, unbelievably, by Marks & Spencer. So much booze. We all wanted to be the last to leave, just as she would have. And everyone was there – parents, aunts, uncles, sisters, half-sisters, and nearly two hundred of our best friends, from almost every stage of our lives, united in celebratory mourning.

And towards the end, after the speeches, after a random, joyous *a cappella* two-step garage choir (of course), after the haunting, plaintive song from her friend David, I stood on the stage, guitar gently weeping round my neck, backed by some of my closest, dearest friends, and we roared through 'Chicago', the whole crowd singing along. There was a balloon drop on the final chorus. And do you know what? Through the tears, through the nerves: we nailed every single last fucking note.

183

The following is a eulogy I wrote for Zarah, printed inside the booklet handed out on the day of her memorial. I didn't have the strength to read it aloud:

Referring to the one we love – the one who makes our world go round – as our 'other half', often seems so informal, so casual and so hackneyed that we can almost flinch. But the more I've thought about it, the more I've come to realise that official alternatives like 'girlfriend', 'partner', or 'fiancée' – they're the casual, throw-away terms.

Because Zarah Harrison, truly, was my other half. She complemented and enhanced me so completely, so utterly, that at times, so right did it feel, that I almost forgot to notice what an exceptional human being she was.

Those epiphanies instead came when she was doing one of her exceptional Zarah-things. Like comforting the girl crying on the Tube. Like giving some of our shopping to the destitute man outside Tesco's doorway. Like making a mere 'party' into an occasion never to be forgotten. Like leaving the party early to comfort a friend whose heart had just been broken. Like cajoling my broken, hungover soul into going to a friend's Sunday birthday lunch 'because we'd promised we would'. Like flaring into sudden anger at the raw human injustice underlying cold, sober news reports. Like comforting me at my lowest moments. Like making me laugh, constantly, always. And above all, inspiring me – and all of us – to try to be like her: to stay in touch with our inner humanity, to value friendship, to never stop enjoying life, and to be the best we can possibly be.

Human history is punctuated by exceptionals, who have walked among us and changed how we see and make sense of the world. Zarah changed the world for each and every person she met, no matter how briefly. She lit up our lives so brightly, so brilliantly, that to have her light extinguished so suddenly, and so early, plunges us into a dimness to which, I suspect, our eyes will take a long time to adjust.

It was never about her, and yet it was always about her. She is irreplaceable – my other. And I am half again.

But, to be sure, I am a better half than before.

The day after the memorial felt like the first day of the rest of my life, but not in any way that I considered positive. Everything was lost. My whole future – our whole future – had been ripped away. It wasn't so much a blank slate as a featureless desert, stretching out to infinity, all familiar landmarks razed to nothing.

Another of grief's paradoxes is that one is simultaneously numb and aflame. I could barely process what had happened to me – to us, to our dreams – and yet was constantly on the brink of tears. At least, when I was awake.

All I could do for the first month or so was curl up and sleep – mainly during the day, with insomnia keeping me awake until the small hours. A paradox, again. 'Downstairs' became almost a foreign country. Friends took turns to sleep in my spare room and keep me company, preventing me from becoming too feral. I embarked on a Herculean late-night task of trying to finish Netflix, and read the whole of Twitter. The concept of 'going out and seeing people' would induce intense anxiety – not just due to the undoubted depression I found myself in, but also due to more practical matters: I was easily tired; I had very little to contribute to any conversation; and the idea of getting a bus or Tube home on my own was too horrible to contemplate. I was fine on my own in the cosy bunkered familiarity of my flat, but being on my own out in 'the real world'… what was the point? Who would I share these experiences with? On one solitary bus journey back to the flat, a homeless man with an enormous dog got on the bus, letting it take up a whole double seat while he sat in the one directly behind. I took a photo to send Zarah. She'd love that. And then I remembered.

'And then I remembered' became an underlying theme. Perhaps the most brutal moments were the few seconds every morning, waking from a dream, turning round in bed to say good morning, to look each other in the eyes… only for reality to crash through. And the dreams… the dreams where the immunotherapy was working, where the scan result was negative, where a multitude of alternate realities would exist… only to be ripped away as I opened my eyes. They never really go away, those dreams.

Throughout this time, thanks to St Joseph's Hospice, I had some fairly intensive bereavement counselling. Steve, my counsellor – a gentle, thoughtful and highly intelligent man who became something of a hero to me – helped me pick through the rubble of my former life, searching for meaning in Zarah's death. And here I stumbled into another of grief's paradoxes: while you simultaneously lose all 'macro' meaning in your life, its place is filled by a thousand micro-meanings.

Everything – every song, every placemat, every keyring, every dog bark, every empty shampoo bottle – suddenly becomes deeply significant, a reminder of your 'previous' life. Everything has meaning. Everything meant Zarah.

And on the horizon loomed a significant event.

It was nearly Christmas.

Although I have always been, and always will be, something of a Scrooge about it, Zarah absolutely LOVED Christmas in a way that had barely changed since she was a child. Over the six years we were together, at her insistence, we'd hosted several wonderful get-togethers for our families, either at rented cottages in Ireland or the UK, or at our flat in London. They were so much fun, she nearly turned me. Nearly.

But now it was time for my first Zarah-less festive period. I didn't want to have to bear it. I *couldn't* bear it. So I did what any sensible mourner would do, and ran away to the other side of the planet.

———

My friend Nettie literally wrote the book on Thailand – she's a former travel guide writer, and hence knows all the country's idyllic isles, postcard sunsets and relaxed, sandy beaches. She'd played a central role in the human safety net I had spent the last few weeks suspended in, and it was her suggestion that three of us – her, me and Lindsey, who, as Zarah's closest friend, was also deeply mired in grief – head to the small Thai island of Koh Lanta, to get away from London and all the Christmas 'cheer'.

It was much-needed. I knew it was time for a break when I found myself stuck in a slow-moving queue in Marks & Spencer, surrounded by a Christmas promotional marketing campaign that Zarah would have undoubtedly had a hand in, as their in-store tannoy blasted out festive pop hits. I'd only popped in because it was on the way home, and had forgotten that seemingly normal things like going into a supermarket could have profound and devastating psychological consequences; I hadn't even thought about M&S being Zarah's previous employers, much less that the sparkling gold yuletide advertising 'signage' would contain echoes of her sparkling gold personality.

As I waited in the slow-moving queue, I could feel my anxiety levels rising, the wave starting to loom, the crest starting to break, downwards towards me. But the real crash came when the tannoy started playing *that* Maria Carey song.

For fuck's sake.

Fully submerged, gasping for air, I placed my basket gently on the floor and ran out of the store.

It was a wintry Friday evening. I arrived at Heathrow's cavernous Terminal 5, clutching my passport, overjoyed to be leaving the country, leaving the flat, leaving my carefully constructed yet increasingly claustrophobic and grotty grief den. A few hours earlier, I'd ceremonially tidied up the flat, ridding it of two months of mouldy takeaway cartons, empty wine bottles and beer cans, and a variety of disposable, no-longer-needed NHS ephemera left over from Zarah's illness. It felt like a small victory – I'd kept my head above water long enough to get to an airport. Now I could get in a real sea, in calm, warm tropical water, and have a break from the protective yet suppressive cocoon that my flat had become. And when I returned, the place would be... different. New. Tidy. Less medical.

Nettie and Lindsey had flown to Southeast Asia two days earlier – I was going to meet them at the airport in Kuala Lumpur and we'd fly to Thailand together. I'd stayed behind because I'd wanted to see the new *Star Wars* film on its first day of release. Because I am, at heart, a massive nerd.

I handed over my passport to the man at the check-in desk: for some reason, I hadn't been able to check in online.

'I'm afraid it's not valid, sir. You'll need a new one.'

'What? Look, it doesn't expire until next year.'

'Yes, May next year. It needs to be valid for six months to enter Thailand.'

I looked at the date on my passport and did the maths. Five months, three weeks and four days. My passport was technically valid, yet because there were three days short of six months left to run, British Airways were refusing to let me on the plane.

'But my girlfriend just died of cancer,' I blurted out, as the waves started to appear on the horizon. 'You have to let me on the plane!' I may have stamped my foot a little bit. I very definitely cried.

'I'm sorry, sir. We might get a fine.'

To cut a long story short, I got the train all the way back to my New, Tidy, Less-Medical grief den, and hid weeping under a duvet for the whole weekend. I emerged on Monday morning, applied for and collected a new 'emergency' passport, travelled all the way back to Heathrow, and got the evening flight to join Nettie and Lindsey on a beach. At least BA had had the generosity not to charge me for the date change. Bastards.

Despite this minor hiccup, Thailand was everything I needed it to be, as I wrapped myself in a warm blanket of sunshine and started, slowly, to heal.

We dived to the bottom of the ocean. We watched the sun set into the Andaman Sea. We ate mountains of barbequed seafood. We took cookery courses. We drank mushroom milkshakes, lay on our backs on the warm sand and watched the clouds turn into fractals. We swam under the moon in the calm, warm phosphorescent waters.

But the significant event, the life-changing moment, the reason I'm telling you this part of the story, came one morning as I lay in bed in a dingy Thai beach hut, reading the Internet on my phone.

I can't recall how, but I stumbled across a link to an article in the *Globe and Mail* – a Canadian newspaper – by a journalist and writer called Christina Frangou. For some reason – perhaps the copy in the social media post that drew me to it – I'd expected to read a piece about a study of suicide rates among people who lose their partners relatively young. What I actually found was so much more – an incredible, heartfelt, personal perspective of her own experience, which, quite unexpectedly, mirrored my own: she herself had lost her partner. In his thirties. To a urological cancer. In a shockingly, brutally short space of time.

In the article – a long-form personal essay about the grief of young widowhood – Frangou sets out in beautiful detail the illness, the hope, the death... and the unbearable little things in her subsequent grief. One section struck me especially deeply:

'I needed to shower. I got out of bed, undressed, turned on the water and stepped in. I spotted Spencer's green bar of Irish Spring soap, resting, partially used, on the edge of the bathtub; its letters had rubbed off weeks ago against his body. I lifted it to my nose. As soon as the scent reached me, I crumpled to the floor of the shower, the smell triggering a flood of memories. That is the smell of our intimacy, of my head on his chest. I curled up with the bar of soap and cried. Then, the dilemma began and I will spend months thinking about this: I have to lather the soap to get that smell. The more I lather, the less soap remains. I hid the soap at the back of the tub, protected from water, and pulled it out on the worst sorts of days. It bubbled into smaller and smaller pieces until, some time in year two, it disappeared down the drain.'

As I lay in bed reading, I slowly, instinctively, curled into a foetal position and began to shake with – 1 don't know what, relief? Sadness? Both, probably. It was like someone had written down my innermost, subconscious thoughts, and published them in a newspaper. The parallels were unreal. There was even, back in my bathroom in London, a half-finished bottle of Zarah's shower gel I'd been slowly eking out since she died.

When I finished reading, I stood up, composed myself… and found something had changed. I felt lighter, like I was at a new stage in the process. I had 'moved on', as they say. OK, only a bit, but it felt tangible. Something in the act of reading that article and realising that my apparently solitary grief was, in fact, something shared, something universal, something fundamentally human… something important had happened. Christina: we haven't met, but thank you. Your writing, your shared experience, literally altered the course of my life.

And that was when I knew: I had to write this book.

I arrived back in London with some semblance of purpose. A book! I had the emails. I had the contacts. I had the medical notes. I had the WhatsApp messages. I had a new insight into cancer. Did I have Something To Say? Ideas began to swirl around in my head. I put out tentative feelers, bouncing the idea off friends.

But, as I retreated into these thoughts, bunkered down in my flat, the waves resumed with a new intensity.

It's hard to characterise what my 'new normal' was like, bobbing adrift in my sea of grief. I noticed, quickly, that a sure-fire trigger for a new deluge was silence – or at least, lack of human noise. The white noise of a morning shower would invariably trigger an avalanche of emotion; the bathroom wall would get a regular pounding almost as fierce as the one meted out in that restaurant bathroom in Cork all those months ago – months that seemed like mere weeks now. So I quickly became addicted to podcasts, and would seldom not have some sort of 24-hour news or talk radio on in the background, whatever the situation, just because the noise would distract me should the Bad Thoughts start up again.

Another paradox: the daily news headlines brought awful tidings from around the world – the global waters were, in their own way, as choppy as my own. I threw myself into them, to escape my own roiling swells by immersing myself in the external. 'How can you bear to listen to it all? It's a never-ending nightmare!' friends would remark. Only relatively, I would say. My inner demons seemed, at the time, fiercer, more malevolent than anything The Donald could muster. And the transatlantic time difference was manna for my insomnia – while the UK was asleep, I was keeping abreast of CNN. On top of this, I felt like I had a duty to be outraged for two: Zarah wasn't here to witness it all – I'd have to be her proxy.

She'd left sketchy, well-hidden instructions for what to do with her ashes. We found them buried in a small green notebook, alongside urology appointment notes and un-done to-do lists – the following shaky, morphine-riddled scrawl:

'Bio-urn. A tree. Not in a cemetery.'

I looked up 'bio-urn' online: it turned out to be a pressed cardboard, biodegradable container with an adaptor at the top for, basically, a plant pot. She wanted to live on in a tree. Very Zarah. But where should we plant her? I had no garden. I was stumped. But I pushed the thought to one side – there were more urgent things to do. At around that time, I'd belatedly opened some of the piles of mail that had accrued while I was in Thailand. And I found a letter, warning me that if I didn't collect her ashes by the end of January, they'd be disposed of.

I checked the date. 30 January. Fuck.

It was a beautiful, calm winter's day when I went, alone, back to the City of London Crematorium to collect her. I walked under the clear blue sky across Wanstead Flats, past the tombs and mausoleums, to the small admin building near the entrance. It was tediously functional. She was surprisingly heavy; I stuffed her into a tote bag I'd brought with me. On the way back to the Tube, I paused at the duck pond, on the side of a small hillock, and watched from afar as a small child and her mother fed the geese and ducks. I rolled up a cigarette – an ex-smoker, I'd very much fallen off the wagon – and chatted to Zarah, in the tote bag beside me.

At home that evening, I ordered the bio-urn, and tucked Zarah into the space next to the sofa, where she remained (no pun intended) for more than a year.

A couple of weeks later, as I sat on my sofa watching the news, the buzzer to my flat went off. 'Delivery,' said the buzzee, via the intercom. I'd noticed the date earlier: Valentine's Day. It would be just like my friends to do something lovely, to try to ease the pain of my first Valentine's Day alone since Zarah died. I eagerly opened the door, as the grinning courier pressed a large package into my hands, assuming, quite understandably, that it was indeed some sort of romantic offering.

As I signed my name on the courier's digital signature widget, I caught sight of the label on the package.

'Bio Urn.'

I bit back a sob. In the background, blaring loudly on the television, the news had turned to the winners of the previous evening's Grammy Awards.

'Hello from the other side,' sang Adele.

I swear I heard a cackle.

Around that time, Florence, Amber and Michael had flown over from Cork for the weekend, to help me and Lindsey with the awful task of sorting through Zarah's stuff.

It took all day. In the end, Florence didn't – couldn't – join in, so completely devastated was she by Zarah's death. It was simply too much for her to go through her daughter's belongings.

We ended up donating at least 10 bin bags of her clothes and shoes to the local charity shop, and donated her make-up and other cosmetics to a women's refuge (What She Would Have Wanted). Several particularly poignant keepsakes were repatriated to Cork. It was devastating, gruelling work, and yet we just got our heads down and did it. Because you have to.

In the middle of all this, while he was going through her files and folders – mainly old bank statements and payslips – Michael found something, and called for me to come upstairs. It was a letter: a report from a bladder cystoscopy that Zarah had had in 2010 – two months before we got together – after yet another painful bladder infection. Although the urologist's conclusion was that things were 'normal', his report described 'patches of inflammation on the upper right-hand side', and recommended she have another appointment at some point later.

The upper right-hand side is, of course, where Tina originated.

I had – I still have – resolved not to play the game of 'what if?' that so consumes people during bereavement, but this made it difficult not to think about what might have happened if those appointments had been made, or attended; it's truly a fool's game. And yet... what might have happened if I'd found that report earlier, as her bladder infections were becoming more frequent, and more painful? Would I have nudged her to go for a scan earlier? Could she have been diagnosed earlier, before Tina had gone on her travels?

Then again, I reminded myself of another counterfactual: the standard treatment for stage 3 bladder cancer is something called a radical cystectomy – a major operation to remove the entire bladder. But in about half of patients who have it, there's a substantial chance the disease comes back later. So there was also a chance that any hypothetical 'earlier' diagnosis would merely have ruined our perfectly happy last Christmas together, and she'd have simply been a cancer patient for longer.

So, like I say, 'coulda shoulda woulda' is a mug's game. Nothing useful would come from that line of thought. Zarah was dead. My girlfriend just died of cancer. Nothing would change that now, and getting involved in a psychological blame-game wasn't going to help anyone.

But the urologist's report also raised another thought in my mind. Had Zarah had cancer the entire time we were together? It would have been the profoundest of tragedies. Coulda, shoulda, woulda… woulda done what, exactly?

These revelations added to the ideas swirling around my head about a possible book. How long had the cancer been there? Was there anything in her tumour data, sitting on a hard drive at the Francis Crick Institute, that might be able to shed light on the idea? The idea of telling the story of Zarah's cancer, as well as of the woman whose life it claimed, started to crystallise.

———

It was a chilly post-Mayday Bank Holiday morning, just six months after Zarah died, when I next went to meet Charlie Swanton at the Crick. Despite the grey, drizzly day, the enormous spaceship-like building still struck awe. I was met in the reception and taken up to the labs by Charlie's PA, Sharon, whom I'd first got to know when she'd worked at an organisation that shared its offices with Cancer Research UK. We gossiped outside his small, glass-fronted office while he finished his previous meeting. 'By the way, I'm so sorry to hear about what happened,' she said, with genuine sympathy and sadness. I was touched.

And yet. Six months on and I still had no answer, no clue how to respond to that, other than a shuffle, a glance at the floor and a muttered 'thanks'.

'Oh, is Henry here? Fantastic. Come on, I'll get you lunch.' As Charlie and I paced through the Institute, he regaled me with a high-speed and captivating anecdote about a trip to see humanity's evolutionary origins during a recent visit to South Africa. Then, over a sandwich in a canteen I feel obliged to describe as 'bustling', I told him where I was heading with ideas for The Book, and how I'd need his help in trying to understand more about Tina. To my huge relief, he was completely taken by the idea, his eyes flashing with characteristic enthusiasm. Another piece of the jigsaw fell in place. He agreed to help in any way, offering his team's expertise in analysing any data from Zarah's tumour that I could get my hands on. The catch, however, was that I'd have to find a way to get the data to him, including that held by AstraZeneca after they analysed Zarah's tumour for the BISCAY study.

Sandwich scoffed, ideas thrown around, we wandered back up to his office, and on the way I mentioned again how much his team's help had meant to me and Zarah. 'It was mainly Nicolai. Have you met Nicolai? You must meet Nicolai.' I had not, in fact, met Nicolai – but we had very briefly emailed each other in August, after Charlie had copied him into an email about the discovery of the amplified *HER2* gene in her tumour DNA, which tentatively suggested that anti-Her2 drugs might be an option if immunotherapy trials hadn't been available.

Back then, desperate but relieved, I'd written to express our gratitude. 'Nicolai, I don't think we've met but I just want to thank you profoundly for your work on this. Fingers crossed for a good response, but just to have this option is incredible.'

He'd emailed back: 'I am truly saddened by your story, but I do hope that what little I, as part of Charlie's team, may have contributed to Zarah's treatment may do some good. This is what our work is all about.'

His reply had, at the time, induced a flood of grateful tears in both Zarah and I. Six months later and Charlie was marching me over to his desk, where he was engrossed in his computer.

Nicolai Birkbak isn't your stereotypical white-coated, pipette-wielding scientist. His lab is in his PC – his field is known as bioinformatics, and involves developing and applying software that can analyse vast quantities of biological information and make sense of the clues it contains. Initially from Denmark, his PhD supervisor had been a mentor and good friend of Charlie's. When Charlie had needed to recruit a data scientist to join his team, Nicolai had jumped at the chance, and moved to London to take up a position at the Crick.

'Nicolai, have you met Henry?' He looked up in surprise from his computer screen, on which was what, from the forest of data on display, I took to be a draft PowerPoint presentation describing Charlie's team's latest findings. After a quick intro, Charlie raced off to another meeting, leaving us with a spectacularly awkward, if happily brief, silence. If the Germans had a word for 'the look on the face of a busy scientist as he unexpectedly meets a man whose dead girlfriend's data he's got saved on his hard drive', I would crowbar it in here. You get the idea.

But if you put two nerds together, you usually get nerdery pretty quickly, and soon we were lost in detailed discussions of intratumour heterogeneity, clonal architecture, and the Swanton lab's latest findings, which had, by some coincidence, been published the previous week, and which my colleagues in the Cancer Research UK media team had, of course, worked on.

Then, out of nowhere, a showstopper. Minimising the slideshow, he clicked on a file in a folder. Four bright-red graphs exploded on to the screen.

'So, this is Zarah's data.'

Fucking hell. Out of the blue, I was looking right into Tina's DNA. The face of the beast herself. Or, more accurately, I was looking into a graphical representation of the degree of genetic chaos in Tina's DNA, the cause of her aggressively lethal rampage through my late girlfriend's body.

Each of the graphs on the screen represented a different sample taken from Tina more than a year ago, just after she'd first made her presence known. Each was further divided into 23 columns, one representing each of the 23 now-scrambled chromosome pairs Zarah had been born with – one of each pair from Z's mother, Florence, the other from her dad, Sean. (I idly, unscientifically, wondered if I could tell which from which, just by looking.)

These chromosomal columns had been annotated according to how far they'd been distorted as the cancer evolved. 'This may seem an odd thing to say to you, but scientifically, this is a really beautiful cancer,' said Nicolai, referring, I surmised, to the cleanness and interpretability of the data. It is not a sentence I'd ever really imagined hearing – my inner geekiness cushioned the words' contradictory blow.

Nicolai pointed to the column representing chromosome 17, and to a tiny spike in the data representing multiple copies of the *HER2* sensor gene. 'That's the amplification. It's relatively small, so our software would normally miss it,' he said. In fact, he explained, seeing data like this – literally seeing it, with eyes, not machines – had led him to rewrite the Swanton lab's analysis software, or 'pipeline'. 'We now use this algorithm, which looks for gaps either side of the *HER2* gene, as well as at the size of the peak, to analyse all our patients' data.'

It took a while for the meaning of this little factoid to sink in. In fact, it didn't really hit me till I got the Tube home after half an hour engrossed in nerd-chat with Nicolai.

Zarah is still helping people. She's still bloody at it. Thanks to a quirk in Tina's DNA, patients on Charlie's future studies will get a slightly more sensitive analysis, which could alert the team to an *HER2* amplification in their tumour's DNA, and mean the patient gets offered targeted drugs that could help them. Because of Zarah. Because of Tina.

I held it together on the Tube, but after I got home the waves, worryingly absent for a few weeks, came crashing back anew. But it was different this time. As well as sadness, there was a new emotion in the mix, one that had been absent for a lot longer: Pride. Pride at how Zarah now also had a legacy – even a little one – in the world of cancer research. Pride at where this research was leading. And in the background, I guess, pride at myself for keeping on with this daft quest.

I put the telly on, made a cup of tea, wiped my eyes, and relaxed back to the normality of Theresa May saying something fucking stupid about Brexit again.

My 40th birthday arrived. I wasn't terribly keen to celebrate still being alive and on my own, but I hired a room in a pub and asked a couple of friends to play some records. It wasn't the all-singing-all-dancing-all-night-all-weekend party that, once upon a time, Zarah and I had begun to plan, but it was something. It was certainly more than sitting in my flat watching Netflix on my own, which was what a large portion of my life still consisted of.

But my friends put on the most extraordinary showing of love and attention – one even wrote and sang a song about me (and yes, Carly, it *was* about me). I'd thought I'd wanted low-key, but this was just perfect. I felt secure, and loved, and – dare I say it – happy.

I want to say something here about my friends – mine and Zarah's friends – because without them I simply wouldn't have progressed so quickly from a shaking wreck of grief to the relatively normal human being that stood in that pub in May 2017. They were my safety net, always there, never outstaying their welcome, always checking in, happy to blow whichever way the wind was blowing me when I wanted to stick my head out of my grief den. For all the terrible luck that had come our way, I am, truly, lucky to have them.

By now, 'the book' was making the transition from nascent idea to actual project – and so my birthday present, from about 30 of them, who all clubbed together to make it happen, was a slick, top-of-the-range laptop, and some travel speakers.

I took them off on a six-week trip across America – a country with which I was now, thanks to my steady insomniac's diet of CNN and politics podcasts, morbidly fascinated. I flew to New York, spent a week bumbling, then headed to DC, then up to see Kieran again upstate, and then the pièce de résistance: I took the train all the way across the country, from New York to San Francisco, via Chicago. It was a trip I'd always wanted to do, but Zarah had steadfastly refused ('Why'd you want to go to America when there are so many other places to go?' she'd said, with ineffable logic).

In San Francisco, I hired a car and struck out by road to a tiny, isolated cabin in northern California.

I holed up there for several weeks. I began to write.

———

It's a chilly November morning, more than a year since Zarah died. Although I've mentally battened down the hatches, the anniversary itself has come and gone without much incident. Writing down your grief, it seems, is a reasonably effective way to cauterise it. Still, the sense of 'this time last year' pervades everything – the plants on the balcony shedding their leaves; the second series of a TV show we'd both loved. The clocks have changed again; the evenings are dark. So near and yet so far.

I arrive at the coffee shop near UCL armed with my notebook and laptop. Pramit is already there, with a colleague who looks after the local tissue repository, where Zarah's samples reside. We're here to discuss exactly what to do with the samples of Zarah's tumour and other material that had been collected over the course of her illness – including nine paired vials of frozen blood and urine that Pramit and Sophia had collected, month by month. A few weeks ago, I had a similar meeting with Charlie and Nicolai at the Crick. It's a game of scientific yin and yang – although the researchers at UCL look after the samples, Charlie's team have the expertise to make sense of the data they contain. In other words, UCL has the treasure, but the Crick has the map.

It's a dark, morbid, but precious treasure. Frozen in these samples, suspended in time, are fragments of DNA shed by the cells of Zarah's cancer as they grew, multiplied and died. The tumour tissue contains layers of information still to be probed. The blood and urine samples represent snapshots, taken at monthly intervals, of what was going on inside Tina herself. Some will have come from the primary tumour in Zarah's bladder. Others may have originated from the cancer cells in her lymph nodes. And later on, in the final couple of samples, there may be fragments from the disease in her liver. Added together, and set alongside other information – scan results, blood tests etc. – they might reveal information about how Zarah's cancer evolved and responded to treatment; about the nature of the mutations that allowed it to spread and avoid the immune system.

If I can find a way to draw all the information together, I might be able to understand why she died; it's also information that could be, in some small way, useful in understanding bladder cancer as a disease, and how to help other people with this horrible condition.

But to do so, there are lots of issues to be resolved. Who will pay for the analyses is a crucial one, as is exactly which analyses to carry out, and which lab will actually do the work.

We part company enthused, but with little resolved.

Later that day, Pramit gets in touch to alert me to another hurdle. The regulations under which Zarah's samples were collected stipulated they must be stored anonymously, only identified by a code number. Deciphering that code, and so allowing Zarah's samples to be accessed, would require navigating the complexities of research ethics bureaucracy. 'We'll find a way round it all,' I reassure Pramit.

And for the first time in ages, I mentally cross my fingers.

———

It's a sunny summer's day in 2018 – more than five years since Annabell's diagnosis – when I sit down with her to interview her for this book. We've become close now – we'd meet up from time to time while I was cocooned in my flat after Zarah died, while everyone else was at work, to watch crap telly and drink tea and chat idly. Two damaged souls, bound together by cancer.

James and I play in a band, too – a part-time phoenix risen from the ashes of Zarah's memorial.

I meet her in London Fields, just up the road from my flat, just down the road from hers and James's.

They've been married a year now. I went to the wedding. It was tough, but so beautiful. One of those days that just radiates warmth, and love, and happiness. And, in the background, less prominently acknowledged, but unignorable: relief.

And of course, for me, sadness too.

I'd nearly lost the plot at the end when, during the inevitable wedding disco, during a particular song – I forget which, but one of Z's favourites – the random Brownian motion of dancing guests, just briefly, caused a gap to open up right in the middle of the dance floor. A gap that, in a parallel universe, would have been occupied by a beautiful blonde extrovert, wearing a big purple dress with a frilly red underskirt, pumping her arms furiously to the music.

It's been, to put it mildly, a tough few years for Annabell as she continued with the immunotherapy, and her tumours continued to shrink. Zarah's death, obviously. Not just the loss of a close friend, but physically seeing Zarah towards the end, in St Joseph's, while she herself still had so many question marks over her future.

And then psychologically readjusting to living, when she'd been convinced she was going to die.

She's still off work, occasionally doing some voluntary work – at a garden, at an 'upcycling' project renovating old furniture, and in a charity shop – while she contemplates what to do next.

But in the main, she's been putting up with the daily grind of chronic, long-term side effects of continued immunotherapy, which she's been taking now, every three weeks, for coming up to 28 months.

'In the beginning, it was sinusitis, which is still a problem now,' she tells me. 'Just constantly having a cold, constantly being blocked up. Every cycle I get some sort of cold, there were just times when it felt like I'd had the flu for months. And then when I finally came off the steroids, it suddenly got worse. And that was when my hearing started going.'

By July 2017, she'd completely lost the hearing in her left ear. No one was sure what the cause was – it could have been a delayed effect from the radiotherapy she'd had to her brain. It could be her hyperactive immune system, or the pembrolizumab itself. Her doctors paused her immunotherapy briefly, but then resumed. Her hearing has continued to deteriorate ever since. She's learned to lip-read.

She's had eczema, and occasional bowel problems. She was diagnosed with an underactive thyroid. She has arthritis too, in her left hip. Sometimes it locks into position while she's asleep. That was a worry initially. Did she want a bone scan? The spectre of the cancer coming back is never far away.

But in the plus column – it seems that, for now, her cancer's vanished. She's a NED – no evidence of disease.

She's at the point of deciding whether to stop taking the immunotherapy. It's a huge decision, one that hinges on a simple question: if the cancer returns, will she be able to start taking it? The hospital's current policy is no. So she continues. As do the side effects.

We talk about Zarah, and I ask about what they talked about, and about the parallels and differences between their experiences of cancer. It's the first time we've ever talked about it properly. She regrets, deeply, I sense, that her own ordeals prevented her from being there more for her friend.

'The sad thing is, even though we both had cancer, we were always in such different places. Occasionally we did have some deeper conversations, and we had points where we were both more with it, but so often, for example, she'd be full of steroids, and really up, and I'd be full of tramadol, and really stoned. But also she had this whole, like "I need to go everywhere, I need to see everyone, I need to make the most of every minute of every day". Which I envied, but I just couldn't do that, that's not how I felt. I had so much else going on. And I feel really sad about that.'

You'd think, wouldn't you, that two close friends, both with cancer, both being treated at the same hospital, would have been bound tightly together by their shared experiences, shared knowledge. But not cancer. Cancer doesn't let you do that. A constantly shifting disease that affects so many, but each profoundly differently. A common enemy that also divides us.

In November that year, several months after I interviewed her, Annabell's hospital changed their policy on immunotherapy. She paused her treatment, with an agreement that she needed to decide by February if she wanted to resume.

In February 2019, she decided to officially stop taking pembrolizumab. For the first time in four years, she was finally free of cancer treatment.

I texted her: 'So pleased for you! How are you feeling? Have you noticed a difference?'

'Not really,' came the reply. 'I've had a nasty infection and further hearing loss issues. But so good not to have to go to Barts all the time though!'

The following month, while she and James were in a pub with some friends, she noticed the conversations around her gradually becoming dimmer. As they left, the last of Annabell's hearing suddenly went. James held her as she kept repeating to him, 'I can't hear. I can't hear anything.' She became completely, profoundly deaf.

Around the same time, during a hospital visit – with James at her side to help convey what the doctors were saying – they noticed her blood sugar was unusually high: she'd developed Type I diabetes – the one where you have to inject yourself with insulin every day.

It was, in James's words, a 'monumentally shitty time'.

'I had to go to every appointment and translate for her,' he remembers. 'I became her secretary and started dealing with all the appointment slots. It was awful for her, as she lost the one thing she had control over – her schedule.'

In June, after months of deafness, Annabell had an operation to have a cochlear implant inserted into her skull. After a few weeks for the implant to bed in, it was switched on, and – just like that – she was able to hear again – a medical miracle on top of a medical miracle.

'So much for stopping the treatment to let my body recover and not have to go to the hospital so much!' she texted.

Despite voluminous quantities of goodwill and good intentions – and many, many emails – it will be nearly 18 months before I finally make progress in pulling together the research data for the book.

It's agreed early on that Mark Linch will lead on coordinating the scientific side of things, while I set off on a mission to find the relevant funding. The researchers involved – Charlie, Nicolai, Mark, Sergio, Pramit, Sophia, et al. – are more than happy to put their time and effort in *pro bono*, but UCL's DNA sequencing machines need more than goodwill to run – and these costs need to be covered. With Mark's support, I approach several funding bodies with a carefully drafted application – alas, the project doesn't fit the criteria, and I'm repeatedly turned down.

Throughout this time, my life starts to move on, returning to something approximating normal. In February 2018, after much soul-searching, I dust off my alarm clock and go back to work. I initially work two days a week, then three, then four – building up, assessing, making sure it's the right thing to do. It's odd being back, and yet comforting. My first few weeks are spent almost literally in one long series of hugs in the corridor, as colleague after colleague welcomes me back. I have a new routine and a new purpose. And this time, as they say, it's personal.

And yet merely writing about cancer isn't enough. I'm restless. I want to DO something about it, as well as writing about people who do something about it. So I start to branch out into the world of what's variously known as patient involvement, patient participation or (slightly awkwardly) consumer involvement – a burgeoning field in which people with experiences of disease are invited to help shape the way the disease's research and care are carried out. I take a voluntary position on a national bladder cancer research committee, and slowly start to chip in to discussions. It's rewarding – but it won't get Zarah's samples analysed, and certainly won't get this book written.

The Book is now a fully developed idea, with a publishing contract in place and, consequently, a deadline. The clock starts ticking. Can I pull this off?

A breakthrough comes – once again – from Charlie Swanton. We meet for lunch in mid-2019, again in the canteen of the Francis Crick Institute. I mention my frustrations in securing funding, the barriers I've been hitting. If there's one thing Charlie can't stand, it's barriers.

'Hold on, I've got an idea.' Charlie pulls out his smartphone and sends an email to a couple of colleagues: it turns out that his team have just started working with a US-based company, ArcherDX, which specialises in analysing the DNA in blood and urine samples. Charlie asks them if they'd consider helping me.

Just half an hour later, we hear back. The company is happy to analyse Zarah's samples.

I feel like crying with relief. And then I do.

In October 2018, on the second anniversary of her death, we planted Zarah's ashes under a cherry tree in a secluded corner of Victoria Park – a little leafy alcove where we'd often gathered for picnics and mischief.

This time, there were no figs to chew on. But we got absolutely smashed in a pub.

It's what she would have wanted.

That was supposed to be the end of this chapter. But cancer's not like that. You should have realised that by now.

In October 2019, almost exactly three years after Zarah died, and as I started to put the finishing touches to this book, it turned out that there was one last, tragic twist to recount.

Almost a year after her last dose of immunotherapy, Annabell had started having headaches and blurred vision, and feeling nauseous. She was having increasing trouble opening her left eye.

Despite her certainty that it was something more sinister, the doctors had initially thought it could be her cochlear implant playing up, or perhaps some late withdrawal symptoms from the immunotherapy.

She spent five days in hospital as they tried to work out the underlying cause. A brain scan appeared to rule out their worst fears. Frustrated, in pain, and not wanting to be in hospital over the weekend, Annabell had gone home. But her condition continued to worsen.

The following week, after repeated calls to the hospital, James managed to book an appointment with her neurological team. When the day came, they were shocked at how quickly her sight had deteriorated, and had another, closer look at the scan taken the week before.

And they spotted something on the scan they'd missed earlier.

Annabell's cancer was back.

And this time, it was inoperable, buried deep in her brain, pressed against one of the nerves that controlled the muscles in her eyes.

Options were limited, but there was still hope: the plan, the doctors had said, was to blast the tumour with radiotherapy to stop it in its tracks, and then try to reverse its growth with a brand-new combination of targeted drugs.

But, once again, cancer said: fuck your plans.

The radiotherapy didn't work – in fact, quite the opposite: it seemed to cause the tumour to start bleeding into her brain. Already spaced out from the painkillers and steroids, nine days after starting treatment, now back in hospital, she lost consciousness completely.

James, together with Annabell's family, who had been at her bedside constantly, were told the absolutely devastating news: that, after all the years of treatment, of the constant struggle, the ups and downs, the cutting-edge therapies, the breakthroughs, the hope, the pain... there was, now, nothing more that could be done but wait. After all her previous tumours had been conquered by chemotherapy, radiotherapy, surgery and immunotherapy, that one single tumour in her brain managed to find a way through.

And in the most bitter, extraordinary twist of fate, when her family heard the news that there was nothing more to be done, Annabell was in the exact same bed in Barts that Zarah had been in, three years earlier, when she was told that her cancer would end her life.

Annabell died, peacefully, on 6 November 2019. Her final diary entry, discovered by James shortly afterwards, reads as follows:

So dear melanoma we meet again.

What news do you bring this time?

A duel you say, oh you have caught me off guard, I was not prepared again.

You are unhappy I scraped through and beat you last time, you have come back stronger.

I, however, was ravaged by the wounds of our last fight and have been slow to bounce back.

This duel may be the last I can summon myself to fight. Beware, tread carefully, for I am reduced to a shadow.

7

Who was Tina anyway?

Z ARAH WAS A HUGE fan of generic 1980s 'whodunnit' TV detective shows – *Poirot, Miss Marple, Murder She Wrote* and the like. She'd while away countless lazy Sunday afternoons glued to episode after episode of repeats, while I pottered around the flat dipping in and out of the (to my mind) endlessly repetitive plots and occasionally hammy acting. And so naturally, while she was ill, stuck at home with plenty of time on her hands as the chemo did its thing, her love for this particular genre of daytime TV reached a new level.

A particular trope (one might say 'cliché') – in such narratives occurs at the finale, as the detective gathers the suspects into a room, and holds court while recapping the evidence, finally to reveal, with a dramatic flourish and much gasping, the murderer's true identity.

So perhaps in tribute to all that, this is the part of the book where I must do my best Poirot impersonation, and assemble all the evidence I've been able to gather about 'whodunnit' – about the molecular and biological events that resulted in Zarah's own death.

I say 'must' – this has been, for me, about more than just solving a biological mystery. Pulling all this information together has been a personal journey of... if not closure, then of trying to understand what happened to Zarah in terms I understand myself. In learning so much about cancer over my career, I've needed to somehow apply that knowledge to answer the inevitable questions anyone who loses someone to cancer has. Why did it happen? When did it start? Could we have done anything to stop it? Could we have stopped her dying? But for me, these questions are, inevitably, reframed in scientific terms. What mutations happened first in her tumour? Which ones came next? Why didn't her immune system spot them? Were there any clues that could have led to better, more sophisticated treatments?

Could we have used these treatments? Would they have worked? How did her cancer kill her?

So as much as what you're about to read should – hopefully – help you understand cancer a bit better, it's also something that, in its writing, has helped me come to some sort of peace with, and understanding of, Zarah's loss, and the fact that – as far as I've been able to determine – no stone was left unturned.

To be able to do this, I've tried to draw together information from a wide range of sources: Zarah's medical records, hard drives at research institutes, talented young researchers' PhD theses, established experts studying bladder cancer, commercial organisations who provide genetic testing for trial participants… and, of course, from tissue, blood and urine samples Zarah donated to UCLH's biobank.

Attempting this has been a monumental task, involving a lot of very busy people going out of their way to help me, and putting up with me pestering them at regular intervals. And it's been an endeavour on which, at several points, for a variety of reasons, I've nearly given up – sheer frustration, bureaucracy, my mental health, the mental health of those around me, to name a few. But alongside these, perhaps the biggest spanner fate threw into my path (he said, mixing metaphors) came right at the end of the process, when I thought I'd overcome them all.

In early 2020, just as I was pulling together the book's final draft, still waiting for the final analyses of various samples to arrive, a new and unsurmountable obstacle appeared. The COVID-19 coronavirus outbreak began, and laboratories around the world – including, of course, those analysing Zarah's samples – ground to a halt. Viruses, it seems, take a similar view of one's plans as cancer does.

Nevertheless, what I was able to pull together, and what you'll read over the following pages, is as complete a picture as I've been able to assemble of the events that occurred in Zarah's bladder.

So let's review the assembled cast of 'suspects' that I've lined up to interrogate.

First, there are the cystoscopy and ultrasound tests, carried out back in 2010, before Zarah and I first met. This, I'd hoped, might yield clues as to how long she'd carried a tumour in her bladder.

Next, there's the DNA analysis carried out on Zarah's tumour, by the team at the Francis Crick Institute, shortly after she was diagnosed.

This information will hold clues as to how – and in what order – Zarah's tumour acquired the 'superpower' mutations necessary to grow inside her bladder and invade the surrounding tissue. But it also may reveal something about what caused these mutations to occur, and so answer the question of what may have caused her cancer in the first place.

I've also been able to draw on work carried out by Mark Linch's team at the UCL Cancer Institute, who included Zarah's samples in their studies of how the immune system reacts to a growing tumour. This work, I hoped, would help me understand why Zarah's tumour escaped detection until it was too late and, potentially, how, and why, it started growing again after her chemotherapy.

Perhaps most intriguing – and arriving just in time for this book's publication, after a long, fraught, COVID-induced delay – is the DNA analysis of six of Zarah's blood samples, taken at regular intervals throughout her treatment. Floating in these samples were tiny fragments of DNA shed by her tumour cells as they grew and died, revealing clues as to how the tumour evolved resistance to chemotherapy. I had nearly given up hope of these ever arriving: quite understandably, in early 2020, as SARS-CoV-2 was spreading rapidly across the world, there were far more pressing matters for clinical researchers to address than this book. Nevertheless, arrive they did.

And finally, I tracked down the analysis of a biopsy sample taken from Zarah's tumour shortly before she died, which may yield more clues about the additional superpowers it had acquired as it grew back after the chemotherapy's onslaught.

In order to explain the detail of what all this means, I'll largely be drawing on scientific concepts I've already discussed in the book – about DNA mutations, the Hallmarks of Cancer, the immune system, and so on. But a quick caveat: there are a few more concepts I'll need to introduce as we go. I'll try to keep it as brief as possible.

But before we get into all this, there are a couple of broader points I want to make.

First, rather than a clear 'whodunnit', what I'm about to describe is what criminal lawyers often refer to as 'the theory of the case' – the available facts assembled into a plausible narrative. Some of this is, of course, speculative. There are, as I've said, a number of facts missing. I have come to accept that I cannot ever know exactly what happened, on a molecular level, in the lining of Zarah's bladder as its cells became progressively more dysfunctional and developed into an aggressively lethal tumour. But such is the state of scientific knowledge about cancer – and in particular, *this* cancer – that I can still make a pretty educated guess.

And second, as you might have suspected, this is a story that you already know – at least in part. Scattered around this book, you'll have read a series of sections describing the fate of a 'mother cell' in the lining of a bladder as it slowly evolves into a monstrous, lethal tumour. I created this story – with a lot of help, from lots of scientists – from the data on Zarah's tumour, which I go into a bit more detail about in this chapter. It depicts, as closely as I can muster, what 'Tina' might have looked like as it developed from a small patch of inflamed cells on the upper right-hand side of Zarah's bladder.

So, with those provisos out the way, let's get into it.

Let's start with a neatly folded letter, dated 10 June 2010 – six years before Zarah's diagnosis, two months before we first met – found among her personal belongings, as four sad individuals – her sister, Amber, her brother-in-law, Michael, her best friend, Lindsey, and me – tearfully cleared out her stuff from our flat.

'Dear Dr Asghar,' it begins. 'Thank you very much indeed for asking me to see this 31-year-old lady with a history of long-standing recurrent urinary tract infections.'

(I can imagine Zarah's hearty cackle at being described as a 'lady'.)

Sent from a consultant urologist to Zarah's GP, the letter goes on to outline, as I briefly mentioned in the previous chapter, the results of two tests – a cystoscopy (i.e. a camera inserted into her bladder) and an ultrasound scan – that Zarah had had, to check her recurrent bladder infections weren't anything more sinister.

According to the letter, the cystoscopy had found patches of 'inflamed-looking' tissue, but otherwise everything appeared normal. Obviously, with hindsight, these could – in theory – be the early signs of cancer.

But, I wondered, was there any way to find out more? Possibly – so I requested the full medical records from the clinic where Zarah had been examined – a process that required Amber to get a Letter of Probate drawn up, then several months of back and forth with the clinic's lawyer to ensure all the necessary confidentiality boxes had been ticked.

The records eventually arrived in my inbox and were, to my non-specialist eye, completely indecipherable – a grainy ultrasound 'movie' that would need specialist interpretation, and some scrawled shorthand, rendered further illegible by grainy digital duplication. Eventually, just before the COVID-19 lockdown began, I sat down with Dr Mark Linch to see if he could help interpret them.

Unfortunately, even Mark's expert eye wouldn't be enough to decipher the ultrasound: this, he said, would need a trained radiologist to properly interpret and, alas, thanks to the cold hand of COVID, it was impossible to find one with time to spare before this book went to print.

But what of the cystoscopy report, and those 'patches of inflamed-looking' tissue on the wall of her bladder it revealed? Could they have been, as I feared, early signs of cancer?

Mark's view was that it was impossible to say. On the one hand, yes, they could. But on the other, they were entirely consistent with the ravages of a bladder infection. The jury was very much out – the available data insufficient to rule either way. My first attempt to play scientific detective on Zarah's tumour had been thwarted.

But let's venture into fantasy for a second, and imagine I were able to invent a time-travel-enabled cystoscope, and use it to go back in time and take a sample from this abnormal tissue.

If I were able to do so, I might be able to ask a researcher to accompany me, and to apply modern analytical techniques – not widely available back in 2010 and, even today, still not used in the diagnosis of bladder cancer – to analyse the DNA from the inflamed cells of the bladder wall. These might reveal whether there were, at that time, any telltale mutations in the cells – mutations that we would one day, years later, find in her tumour. And this would tell us whether, in August 2010, just months after these tests, when I first met her, eyes sparkling, dressed as a pirate, in the queue to a music festival, Zarah already carried a proto-tumour in her bladder.

And, armed with such knowledge, hypothetical past-me might be able to do something about it.

But, alas, I do not have a time-travel-enabled cystoscope. I try not to let this frustrating line of thought haunt me too much.*

———

The next, and perhaps most important, piece of evidence on which my case rests is the analysis of the genetic chaos in Zarah's bladder, carried out when she was diagnosed in January 2016. This is the multi-region 'turducken' DNA analysis that Charlie Swanton, Nicolai Birkbak and their colleagues carried out at the Francis Crick Institute, which I initially outlined on pages 58–60 of chapter 2.

At the time I first spoke to Charlie about what they'd found, early in Zarah's illness, I'd only really cared about one thing: whether her tumour had an Achilles heel – a ubiquitous mutation, found in every tumour cell, that might confer some sort of vulnerability, and so suggest ways to help her.

His answer, at the time, had been a tentative 'no' (with one exception: he'd suggested that the tumour *might* be sensitive to drugs targeting a particular amplified gene – drugs that were, and still are, unproven in bladder cancer).

What, then, did Charlie's team's analysis reveal about Zarah's tumour, and the forces that shaped it?

Unsurprisingly, Zarah's tumour was not a 'typical' bladder tumour. Bladder cancer is a disease occurring most commonly among older people (mainly men), often with a history of smoking, and whose tumour DNA – thanks to decades of exposure to toxic, DNA-damaging carcinogens as they drain through the bladder – is often riddled with

*An added, parenthetical, complication now emerging from scientific research is that, even if I'd been able to have this hypothetical, time-travelling test carried out, it would, almost certainly, reveal the presence of a handful of suspicious-looking mutations in the cells of Zarah's bladder – *regardless of whether she had cancer or not*. This may seem incredible, but it's now being discovered that *all* of us, as we age, become a patchwork quilt of millions of slowly growing proto-cancers. The unfolding, deeper paradox – ironic, given the stories I've told in this book – is why the development of cancer is so *incredibly rare* among the billions of cells that make up our bodies, rather than why it is so common among the human population – who all, of course, die of *something*. But I digress.

mutational spelling mistakes, and composed of many distinct groups (or subclones) of cells. In fact, bladder tumours are generally among the most highly mutated, diverse tumours – third, behind lung cancers and melanoma skin cancers.

But Zarah was in her 30s when her tumour developed and, at worst, an occasional social smoker. So, instead, rather than thousands of DNA-scrambling mutations, the cells of Zarah's tumour each carried just a couple of hundred such errors – an order of magnitude lower than usually found in bladder cancer. This is still a lot of damage – and remember it can take just one letter of difference in the DNA code to cause profound problems (just ask anyone with sickle cell disease). But as far as bladder cancer goes, a 'mutational burden' (to use the scientific term) of just 200-odd spelling errors suggested that, whatever caused Zarah's cancer to develop, it wasn't years of exposure to a directly DNA-damaging chemical.

Instead, this relative normality – in terms of single-letter mutations – belied a deeper chaos.

When Charlie's team looked at the overall state of Zarah's tumour's chromosomes, it was not a pretty picture. Whole sections, containing scores of vital genes, had been duplicated, often many times over. Other chunks of DNA were missing entirely, deleting vital genes from the cell's sophisticated and finely balanced control systems. This disastrous situation is found frequently in other forms of cancer, such as breast cancer and some types of bowel cancer, and seems to originate when cells' own DNA replication and repair systems are somehow compromised, causing them to stammer and stutter when copying or repairing their DNA as they gear up to dividing in two.

So, rather than typos in individual words, Zarah's tumour was characterised by scores of copy-and-paste errors, in entire paragraphs and pages of her personal book of life. This suggests that, from relatively early in its development, her tumour was driven, at least in part, by internal forces of instability – of erroneous repair and replication – rather than by external assault.

Charlie's analysis found another level of gross abnormality too, reinforcing this picture. Each cell in her tumour, rather than containing 46 chromosomes as is the norm, carried *double* that amount: 92 entire chromosomes, each of which was riddled with copy-and-paste gene-duplication errors. This suggests that, at some point in the tumour's development, a single dividing cell had somehow failed to separate its chromosomes into two. The result: a monstrous, unwieldy offspring, carrying twice the genetic material of a normal human cell. A spare copy of life's manual, each able to be scrambled in parallel.

So much for the errors on a cellular level. What about variation between cells in different regions of the whole tumour? Was it, to hark back to my earlier gastronomic metaphor, a three-bird turducken? A monstrous Fearnley-Whittingstall-inspired ten-bird roast? Or just a regular, if somewhat mutant, chicken? This next bit might get a bit convoluted, but don't worry, there are a couple of diagrams to help make sense of it all.

Charlie's team had analysed DNA extracts from four separate tumour samples, from physically distant regions of the alien mass growing in Zarah's bladder. Each of these was composed of millions of individual cells, each with its own scrambled genome.

The first region they looked at seemed to be made up of cells with just two distinct genomes. Let's call these groups A and B.

The second sample also contained group-A cells, but also a third, different group, which we'll call C.

The third sample contained all three types of cell – mainly type B, but also traces of cells from both the A and C groups.

And the final sample was also mainly group B, plus a few C cells, but a handful of a new, fourth type: D.

By comparing the genetic characteristics of these different populations of cells – A, B, C and D – Charlie's team was able to work out how they were related to each other, and thus in which order they arose.

Group A, B and C's cells contained all the mutations found in the cells of group D, but each also contained a handful of extra mutations. This suggested that group D's cells were part of a single clump of cells, out of which A, B and C subsequently evolved and grew out. On top of this, none of the extra mutations in group A's cells were present in cells from either B or C – so group A arose out of D separately.

Similarly, group C's cells contained all of the DNA errors present in group D, but none of the additional mutations from group A. It too must have arisen as a descendent of group D.

Group B, however, contained all of group C's faulty genes (and hence, all of group D's), but also a few unique mutations of its own, and none characteristic of group A. This strongly suggested that group B was

FIGURE 2 Cell composition of four samples taken from Zarah's tumour at diagnosis

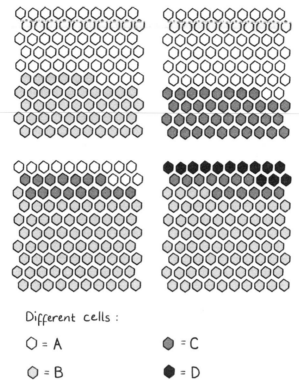

Different cells :

O = A   ◐ = C

◔ = B   ● = D

Genetic analysis showed four different types of cancer cell, present in different amounts in different samples. Most of the tumour is made of three groups - A, B and C. Group D cells were present in lower amounts.

descended from group C, after the latter had itself arisen from the ancestral group D – the 'trunk' of its evolutionary tree:

It's hard to convey how I felt when I was first shown the tree diagram of Zarah's tumour, on a folded bit of paper, over coffee in the canteen of the UCL Cancer Institute, about a year or so after Zarah's death. It was an odd mixture of deep fascination and intense sadness. I remember wondering: am I the only human on Earth with such a profound understanding of the molecular origins of his own grief? OK, that's perhaps fanciful, and certainly a little hyperbolic... but it was, truly, surreal.

Let's turn now to the genetic mutations themselves. What gene faults were present in the different groups of cells in Zarah's tumour? And what do they suggest about how it developed?

FIGURE 3 Evolutionary relationship between cell types in different tumour samples

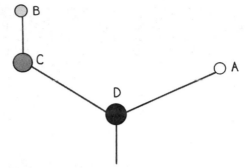

Cell group 'D' is the originating clone, out of which 'A' and 'C' evolved. Group 'B' cells subsequently arose out of group 'C'.

Let's start with the cells of group D, and two critical genes in particular. Their ubiquity in all the samples suggests that they are among the earliest, and therefore most important, events in her tumour's development, found in every copy of its genome analysed – both group D and its descendants, A, B and C.

One gene is known scientifically as *CDKN2A*, the other as *TP53*. Both are well-known culprits when it comes to cancer, so let's discuss each in turn.

The acronym CDKN2A stands for 'Cyclin-Dependent Kinase iNhibitor 2A', and it's a gene that makes a protein whose job is to regulate the activity of another type of protein, called a cyclin-dependent kinase. And these cyclin-dependent kinases activate a third type of protein, one that is absolutely critical to a cell's ability to divide, known as a cyclin.

I suspect your head is spinning slightly, so I'll cut to the chase. *Cyclins are the vital proteins that tell cells when to divide.* They were first discovered in the 1980s, by a British researcher called Tim Hunt. Around the same time, another young researcher, Paul Nurse, discovered their partners – cyclin-dependent kinases – which activate the cyclins, triggering cell division. Both Nurse and Hunt would win Nobel Prizes for their work, and the latter would end up as chief executive of Cancer Research UK – a job he was carrying out rather successfully when I joined the charity in 2003.

But I digress, so let's recap: proteins called cyclins control whether a cell divides, and others – cyclin-dependent kinases, or CDKs – control the activity of cyclins themselves. But there is a third level of control to all this: yet *another* family of proteins, which prevent CDKs from letting cyclins trigger cell division, and so make sure a cell only divides at precisely the right time. These are called cyclin dependent kinase inhibitors, or CDKNs. It turns out that one of them is particularly important in regulating the slowly dividing cells in the lining of the bladder, and it's made using instructions encoded in the *CDKN2A* gene I mentioned above. Charlie Swanton's analysis showed that, very early in the development of what would become her tumour, both copies of its instructions were *completely deleted* from the DNA of a single cell in Zarah's bladder. This, in fact, is the 'control switch', whose loss I described in the second 'sci-fi section' on pages 12–14.

The complete deletion of *CDKN2A* from a cell's genome is – it transpires – relatively common in bladder cancer (and a number of other cancers), and likely has the effect of relaxing the conditions under which cells can divide. It's not, in and of itself, a catastrophe – but it *is* something that allows the cells to grow faster, replicate more often, and, well, just become a bit cancer-y. Hence, I'm choosing to pick it out of our metaphorical whodunnit line-up, and propose that this was one of the first, most important events in the development of Zarah's tumour.

The second gene I want to focus on is known as *TP53* – an absolutely remarkable, evolutionarily ancient gene, found in pretty much all complex life, whose importance in cancer is so profound that entire books have been written about it. I won't attempt to recount its full story here.

In Zarah's case, the situation with *TP53* turned out to be complex. The Crick team's analysis of her tumour revealed that a cell growing in her bladder had picked up a particularly interesting (read: nasty) mutation in each of its two copies of the *TP53* genes (you'll remember that each of our cells carries two copies of every chromosome, and thus every gene it bears: one from each of our parents).

But before we get to that, I need to explain what the *TP53* gene 'normally' does.

Found on a short stretch of DNA on human chromosome 17, *TP53* encodes the instructions for a metaphorical 'Swiss army knife' protein, known as p53, that carries out a variety of functions in our cells. Viewed in the round, its combined abilities make it the master regulator of a cell's fate – indeed, it is often grandiosely referred to as the Guardian of the Genome, preventing cells from accumulating the sort of damage that, if left unchecked, could snowball into a cancer.

The detail of how it does this in practice is extraordinarily complex, with much still unknown (despite decades of research). But broadly speaking, it has two distinct modes of action.

If a cell accumulates relatively minor damage, its p53 proteins trigger a cascade of events that cause the cell to pause, take stock, and try to fix whatever issue ails it. It seems to invoke a sort of stasis, buying a cell time to correct whatever troubles have befallen it.

On the other hand, if the damage is more serious – or cannot be repaired – p53 triggers the cell's built-in death mechanisms, including suicide by apoptosis (see pages 43–44 for a recap). If you've ever been sunburnt (and who hasn't?), you'll have felt p53 at work, tripping the apoptotic switch in your skin cells, causing them to die in the aftermath of the sunlight's assault.

As you might imagine for such a powerful damage sensor, the *TP53* gene is found to have been deactivated or deleted in more than 50 per cent of cancers – including the majority of bladder cancers.*

Since its discovery in the late 1970s (by Professor Sir David Lane – another Cancer Research UK alumnus), decades of research have revealed an almost unfathomable amount about how the *TP53* gene, via the p53 protein it encodes, protects us from cancer. But for all these decades of research, and despite the fact that about 11 million people a year around the world die from p53-deficient cancers, researchers have so far failed to come up with a therapy that specifically targets them. This might seem extraordinary and is, you may note, in sharp contrast to the many recent drugs that target cancers with overactive genes like *EGFR* and BRAF (as discussed in chapter 2) – the vemurafenibs, trastuzumabs, imatinibs and others like them.

In part, this is because it turns out to be far easier to design molecules to switch hyperactive genes *off* than it is to *reactivate* processes that have become disabled or deactivated. But it's also testament to the profound complexity of p53, and its place at the heart of life's control mechanisms.

Back to Zarah's *TP53* mutation. The Crick team identified a single SNV spelling mistake – T instead of a C – that had caused its instructions

---

*There are even poor folks who are born with an inherited defect in the gene, and have to live with a condition called Li-Fraumeni syndrome, leaving them with a greatly increased lifelong risk of cancer.

to be garbled, causing the replacement of one amino acid, arginine, with another, tryptophan, in the resulting p53 protein. Known as an R282W mutation, it's relatively under-studied compared with other p53 mutations, but it seems that, as well as causing p53 to *lose* several of its essential abilities – notably its ability to flip the apoptosis suicide switch – this mutation confers the p53 protein with extra functions, allowing it to *activate* various cellular programs as well. These programs appear to include one (known scientifically as the 'epithelial-mesenchymal transition') that makes cells more likely to spread, and another that's essentially a cellular detoxification system, allowing it to break down toxins like cancer drugs. None of this is good news – it's rare, but people with cancers bearing this mutation appear to do worse than those with more common *TP53* errors.

Zarah was exceptionally unlucky to start with, but to have developed this particular uncommon DNA fault was an extra layer of tragedy heaped on top.

To further compound this bad luck, at some point in the tumour's early development, a single *TP53* mutant cell had picked up a much more serious defect in its remaining normal copy. To repair the damaged region, the cell had no option but to use the mutated, cancer-promoting copy as a template, thus hard-coding the mutation into both chromosomes.

So, putting all that together, Charlie's team found – among several mutated genes – that these two key cancer-preventing proteins were lost or damaged in the early development of Zarah's tumour: the *CDKN2A* cell-division regulator, which had been somehow deleted in its entirety, and the *TP53* genome guardian, which had been scrambled into a defective yet hyperactive form, simultaneously accelerating its growth and rendering it resistant to apoptosis, and also allowing its genome to become more and more disordered and unstable.

Resistance to apoptosis; ability to grow unchecked; unstable genome; potential to spread… one by one, you can see Weinberg and Hanahan's Hallmarks of Cancer (see pages 41–48 for a recap) starting to be sketched out, in four-letter code, in Zarah's very DNA.

Which of these events happened first, we'll never know. The data can't even, really, say for sure that they were indeed defining events – although it's highly likely that they were. All we can conclude is that they both happened, one after another, in an early ancestor of all the cells that made up the tumour that grew in Zarah's bladder, which eventually spread around her body and killed her.

What is clear, however, is that both events happened prior to a separate, equally crucial event in the timeline – one that I mentioned earlier: the doubling of the cell's entire genome, leaving it with twice the usual amount of genetic material. This doubled genome, again present in every cell Charlie's team analysed, carried the rogue *TP53* gene in quadruplicate, and completely lacked any copies of the *CDKN2A* gene. It would have been incredibly unlikely for each of these gene errors to have happened twice, so the data suggests that the genome doubling happened afterwards.

This doubling event itself is significant – while in itself it may not have had a huge effect on the behaviour of the cells containing it (and their descendants) beyond causing them to grow somewhat faster, in evolutionary terms it is hugely important. It provided an entirely new substrate upon which natural selection could act: a parallel genome, able to evolve separately, accruing new errors and deletions to fuel the tumour's subsequent growth.

There are a few more curios to mention. Along with the loss of *CDKN2A* and the mutation of *TP53*, Charlie's team identified a few other genes that were also ubiquitously damaged or missing in Zarah's tumour – genes that have cropped up in large catalogues of cancer-linked genes available to researchers. Their presence, and persistence, in Zarah's tumour is therefore strong circumstantial evidence that they were also part of the problem. Among these genes, one jumps out of the data, one that I mentioned earlier in the book, and which is worth dwelling on: *HER2*.

We first met *HER2* in chapter 2. It makes a protein called HER2, which functions as a tiny 'antenna' on a cell's surface, conducting growth signals from its exterior. It's the target of several cancer drugs, most notably trastuzumab (better known as Herceptin), and is well-known to researchers and clinicians as a 'breast cancer' gene, since it is often found to be repeated many times over (or 'amplified') in the DNA from breast tumours (hence the widespread use of Herceptin to treat that disease).

Zarah's tumour DNA carried some form of amplification of the *HER2* gene – in other words, while the gene itself was 'normal', it had been duplicated over and over, so many copies were now present, joined end to end along each chromosome, allowing it to produce abnormally high levels of the HER2 protein, 'amplifying' its effects. This event seems – according to one reading of events – to be present in all the cells in her tumour.

But there's a quirk in the data that suggests this may not have been the case, that it may not have been a 'trunk' mutation: its amplification seems far smaller than usually occurs in breast cancer – just three or four extra copies, compared with tens or even hundreds.

So there are two possible explanations. On one hand, it could be exactly what it seems: that every cell in Zarah's tumour contained a short amplification of *HER2*, causing it to become extra sensitive to growth signals. But there's another option, also consistent with the data: the existence of a small subset of cells containing a more typical, more extensive, breast cancer-like amplification of many hundreds of copies, whose signal has been 'drowned out' by their non-amplified neighbours.

The data are equivocal, and I've had a bit of debate with Charlie, Nicolai and Mark Linch about which way to call it. These are the sorts of fuzzy, debatable data on which real, life-or-death clinical decisions can be made. There was a point in Zarah's illness where it looked like trying to get hold of some Herceptin-like drugs was a possibility (although their usefulness in bladder cancer is still unproven). In the end, we went for the immunotherapy option, and we'll never know whether targeting the HER2 proteins in her tumour might have blocked its growth. In the first scenario, it might have worked well – if the *HER2* mutation was in the 'trunk' of Tina's evolutionary tree, these drugs might have been quite effective. In scenario 2 – a small subclone of HER2-bearing cells – it may have been far less effective. Who can say? But I hope it illustrates an important point: that deciding on treatment options using tumour DNA sequencing is still *really hard*, even with a team of world-class researchers and clinicians making them.

Now, there are two other elements of the Crick's analysis of Zarah's tumour that I want to discuss before we move on.

The first is the presence of what are known as 'mutational signatures' – fingerprints, left in the DNA code, of different processes at play as a tumour develops. These manifest as particular patterns of DNA changes across a cancer's entire genome, and researchers have now identified more than 30 discrete patterns of DNA alteration – each representing the fingerprints of a different biological process at play in a tumour's history. Of these 30 patterns, culprits have been pinned down for 16.[1] The remainder are, at the time of writing, still a mystery.

One of the patterns that *is* well understood, and seen frequently in DNA from melanoma skin cancers, is characterised by a run of two cytosines (the letter 'C' in the DNA alphabet) being converted to two thymine 'T's. This is exactly the sort of DNA damage observed by laboratory researchers after exposing DNA to ultraviolet light. Its existence in melanoma proves beyond doubt that excessive sun exposure causes skin cancer.

Other signatures correspond to other well-known biological processes, such as the action of various tobacco carcinogens, environmental toxins, or in-built DNA repair processes. A particularly common one appeared to be due to an 'exposure' that none of us can do much about: the natural decay of our genomes as we grow older.

So what did the Crick's data have to say about the processes that shaped Tina's development? Was there anything that might point the finger at what 'caused' Zarah to develop cancer?

The main stumbling block in unpicking these mutational signatures is something I discussed earlier: Zarah's tumour had relatively few mutational 'spelling mistakes' from which to deduce them. But the data did show what Nicolai called 'weak evidence of APOBEC activity'.

'APOBEC' stands for 'apolipoprotein B mRNA editing enzyme, catalytic polypeptide-like', but you don't really need to know that. What you *do* need to know is that APOBECs are nature's antivirus software – a family of related, evolutionary ancient proteins made by our cells, whose members all possess the ability to induce mutations in viral DNA or RNA, preventing themselves from being infected.

They all seem to work similarly, homing in on viral DNA or RNA, attaching to it at specific sequences, and chemically scrambling its code in a way that leaves behind particular signatures of mutations.

It was these signatures that unexpectedly cropped up as researchers started analysing the mutational patterns in tumour DNA. It seems, quite incredibly, that one of the key drivers of cancer in humans is our own antiviral defences – our APOBEC proteins, inside our own cells, becoming inappropriately activated, and causing catastrophic damage to our own genomes.

I remember the first time I learned about this concept, I was gobsmacked. We cause our own cancer, *by mistake*.

Exactly why this should happen at all is still unknown, and there are many theories kicking around. Most prominent, but far from nailed down, is the idea that the chaotic DNA of rapidly dividing cancer cells forms tiny loops of DNA, which 'look' like viral DNA to our APOBEC virus software; it attacks; catastrophe ensues.[*]

According to Nicolai, and others I've spoken with, the DNA data from Zarah's tumour contains fairly convincing evidence that at least some of the damage was caused by her own APOBEC antivirus software – and that this was an ongoing process, occurring, perhaps sporadically, throughout the progression of her disease. And so to the final concept, and evidence, from the Crick analysis I want to touch on. It involves the immune system, and the idea of neoantigens.

You'll remember, from chapter 3, that a 'neoantigen' is the generic name for any abnormal, mutant protein a tumour produces, that can be recognised by the immune system. You might also remember that Charlie Swanton's team – working with Mark Linch – had offered to scour Zarah's tumour DNA for potential mutations that might have caused it to make neoantigens. And if they found any, potentially to go fishing in her tumour samples for immune cells that might recognise them. And if all that were possible, they would try to multiply these immune cells into a groundbreaking anti-cancer treatment.

Obviously, that didn't pan out – this would be a very different book if it had.

But what did happen? Did Zarah's tumour, in fact, produce any neoantigens? And what can this tell us about how it developed, and the processes shaping it?

---

[*]Another theory suggests that APOBECs become activated by the low-level inflammation that builds up as a tumour starts growing – inflammation that might look like a viral infection. Neither of these, you'll note, is mutually exclusive; there's evidence for both, and both may well happen simultaneously. But here's another interesting observation: APOBEC signatures are particularly common in cervical cancer, which is caused by the human papillomavirus (HPV), suggesting that the virus itself is activating APOBEC in this form of the disease. Could other – as yet unidentified – viruses be triggering cancer in humans? It's a compelling, if somewhat speculative, idea. Whatever the reason, I suspect that figuring it out will be just as big a milestone in cancer research as the discovery of p53, or PD-1, or BCR-Abl, or any of the others we've touched on in this book.

Predicting whether a given DNA mutation will generate a protein that the immune system can recognise is still a science that's in its infancy. It relies largely on software algorithms that look at actual DNA sequences, convert them to hypothetical amino-acid sequences, and look at these for patterns that have been shown, in the lab, to cause an immune response. It's complex, experimental stuff.

But let's go back a step. Zarah's tumour contained a relatively low number of 'spelling mistake' mutations, meaning it's unlikely that it made many neoantigens. This is much less than a 'typical' bladder tumour, which generally contains thousands of mutations, and thus far more possible neoantigen candidates. I spoke with Mark Linch and Sergio Quezada – Mark's immunologist colleague at UCL Cancer Institute – about this. Their assessment, after running Zarah's tumour DNA through their experimental prediction software, was that there were 'only a handful' of likely potential neoantigens, only a few of which resided (conceptually speaking) on the tumour's evolutionary 'trunk' (and so present on all its cells).

But 'only a handful' isn't 'none' – so the tumour might have been 'visible' to *some* degree. Just evidently not enough to trigger a full immune assault.

In fact, Mark and Sergio were briefly – in late summer 2016 – able to isolate a solitary T-cell from a sample of Zarah's blood that seemed to be able to recognise one of the hypothetical neoantigens predicted by Charlie's software. For an extraordinary moment, it looked like an experimental, world-first therapy might be on the cards. But his team was never able to replicate this finding. And then things for Zarah moved downhill rather rapidly. It always was the longest of long shots.

Experimental therapies aside, this mere handful of neoantigens provides a partial explanation of how 'Tina' remained hidden from Zarah's immune system in the first place. But explaining the other reason requires me to bring in some good old-fashioned Darwinism, and the concept of 'selective pressure'.

It's time for a thought experiment.

Consider a dividing ball of cancer cells, surrounded by immune cells that are poised and ready to attack. Let's assume that, at the start of this thought experiment, these cancer cells bear no neoantigens – they can continue to multiply, and accrue new mutations at random, in peace. Now consider what happens should one of these cells develop a mutation that allows it to grow faster, but also generates a neoantigen: the immune system will immediately spot it and eliminate it. But if the mutation is 'helpful' to the tumour, yet *doesn't* produce a neoantigen, the immune system will ignore it. Effectively wearing an invisibility cloak, this new subclone can rapidly outgrow its competitors and, eventually, replace them.

This is classic evolution by natural selection. In Darwinian terms, the immune system is a 'predator', and the tumour its 'prey'. Over time, the immune system shapes a tumour's evolution by eliminating cells that develop obvious neoantigens, while allowing 'hidden' growth-promoting mutations to arise.

Evidence supporting this idea of an evolutionary arms race, between tumour and immune system, is building all the time. Data emerging from Charlie Swanton's mammoth TRACERx programme – studying people with lung cancer as they progress through the disease – is just one example.[2] Time and time again, tumour DNA analyses show evidence of what is now called 'immuno-editing' – the immune system's systematic pruning of a tumour, ridding it of neoantigen-bearing cells while allowing others to grow unhindered. A malign twist on Darwin's fundamental principles.

So, let's pull together everything we have so far, and use the Crick analysis to paint a scientific picture of what was growing in Zarah's bladder by January 2016, when she first went to A&E in Cork with a 'kidney infection'.

It seems that Zarah's tumour started from a cell in her bladder that, for reasons unknown and probably due to random bad luck, developed several key catastrophic features one after another: most importantly, the loss of both copies of its *CDKN2A* growth suppressor, and then, later, its *TP53* genome guardian. This cell grew into a tiny, uniform mass of cells, still more or less invisible to the immune system. As these cells grew, their DNA became disordered, thanks, in part, to the loss of the p53 guardian protein. And this, somehow, triggered their APOBEC proteins to start to carve up their genomes at random. Most of these resulting mutant cells died – either because of the catastrophic genomic errors, or perhaps because they began producing neoantigens, alerting the immune system. Eventually, one cell within this small, growing mass failed to divide properly and duplicated its entire genome, allowing it to grow slightly faster than its neighbours. And then one of *these* cells acquired an amplification of one copy of its *HER2* genes, causing it to grow even more rapidly, to further out-compete its neighbours, who slowly receded in number.

Finally, these millions of rapidly *HER2*-driven growing cells then diversified – perhaps, again, due to APOBEC activity – into at least three separate clones of cells, all still invisible to the immune system, to form an enormous mass that practically filled her bladder. And all of this hive of catastrophic cellular activity went entirely unnoticed by Zarah, until the mass grew big enough to block the entrance to her bladder.

It sounds so cold and clinical to describe it like that – but by now you've read the other side of the story too, and the awful human consequences of this molecular, cellular Darwinian corruption.

Now, before we move on to the next section, a brief caveat. At the time she was diagnosed, the tumour in Zarah's bladder was enormous – enough to take up almost its entire volume, and composed of billions of cells. By comparison, the samples the Crick team analysed were tiny. It is possible that what we've called the 'common ancestor cells' of all the other groups – 'group D' in the diagram we saw earlier – was itself a descendent of another group of cells, resident elsewhere in the tumour, and un-analysed – and that what we are calling the 'trunk' of the tree is, in fact, a mere branch. It might be that there were other clones of cells, with other hallmarks, in other regions of her tumour, carrying other 'hallmark' mutations, that would undermine the exact facts, if not the broad trajectory, of this narrative.

But all that said, this is the best we've got to go on – and it will have to do for now.

So let's now turn our attention outwards, from the tumour's internal genomic chaos, and look at what Mark Linch, together with Pramit Khetrapal and Sophia Wong – the two junior doctors turned cancer researchers whom we befriended as they collected Zarah's blood and urine for their PhD projects – were able to learn about how her immune system tried, and failed, to tackle the monster in her bladder, both as it grew, and as it adapted as she was given the chemotherapy.

———

What follows is almost entirely the hard work of Mark's PhD student, Sophia, and I owe her a huge debt of gratitude for allowing me to use her work in this book. It's also worth noting that Sophia's decision to focus her PhD on bladder cancer had come about by accident. She'd initially planned to focus on prostate cancer, but there happened to be a dearth of blood and urine samples from such men at UCLH. Helpfully, Mark had suggested that, to refine her immunology techniques while she waited for suitable samples to arrive, she 'practise' on samples collected from a recently diagnosed bladder cancer patient.

That patient, of course, was Zarah.

Sophia began working with two sources of Zarah's biological material: tissue samples taken from Zarah's tumour at diagnosis; and the blood and urine samples she donated to them, every few weeks, as she went through treatment.

Let's start with what she learned from the tumour itself, using a technique called immunohistochemistry, which allows different types of immune cell in a tissue sample to be seen down a microscope.

Sophia discovered that Zarah's tumour, at the time she was diagnosed, contained three separate types of T-cell. There were large numbers of cytotoxic T-cells – the hand-to-hand soldiers we met in chapter 4, which are the crucial immune cells that combat cancer. Also present were so-called helper T-cells – the generals that help marshal and coordinate an immune response.

But Sophia also saw large quantities of a type of T-cell called a 'regulatory' T-cell. These are known to shut down the activity of other immune cells, to stop an immune response from spiralling out of control.

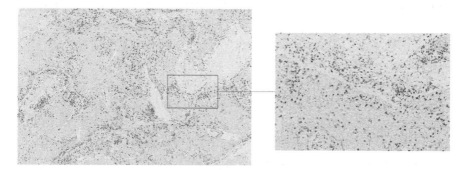

A sample of Zarah's tumour viewed down a microscope, treated so that the different types of T-cell are visible.

It seemed that Zarah's tumour had indeed tripped some sort of alert mechanism, calling in the cytotoxic and helper T-cells to try to eliminate it. But somehow, circumstances had conspired to also call in the regulatory T-cells, switching off the anti-tumour immune response and allowing the tumour to continue to grow unchecked.

Let's turn now to Zarah's blood and urine samples, and the immune cells in them. These capture – for the first time in this story – what happened *after* her diagnosis, after she started chemotherapy, and her tumour became resistant to it.

Shortly after Zarah began chemo – during her second cycle – Sophia visited us in the ward. She'd been studying the levels and activity of the T-cells in Zarah's blood, and had a question: had Zarah had a cold or flu since her previous chemo?

She hadn't. Sophia looked excited at this response.

She went on to explain what had prompted her question: she'd spotted a sudden jump in the level of cytotoxic T-cells in Zarah's blood – suggesting that *something* had activated her immune system.

If it wasn't a viral infection then it suggested that, perhaps, in response to the chemo, Zarah's cytotoxic T-cells were finally waking up to the monster in their midst, and, perhaps, overcoming the repression imposed by the regulatory T-cells. It was, at the time, very encouraging news to hear – a small ray of hope shining through the gloom. Could this, perhaps, be signs of something more profound: a strong immune response, triggered by the chemotherapy, that might hold Zarah's tumour at bay for a considerable time? We had dared, gently, tentatively, to hope.

But as time went on, and Zarah and I eagerly asked Sophia 'how the T-cells were doing' during Sophia's regular trips to meet us after appointments at UCLH, Sophia became slightly cagier.

I would only understand why much later.

Over months, Sophia had carefully tracked the levels of T-cells in Zarah's blood and urine, and their degree of activity. Up and up they went, becoming progressively more active as the chemo blasted her tumour.

After three cycles of chemotherapy, Sophia had spotted more hints that Zarah's immune system was starting to gain the upper hand against her tumour. The number of T-cells in her urine had gone down, which, in studies of other patients with bladder cancer, had been a positive sign. Also, in samples of Zarah's blood that had been sent to a laboratory in

Denmark, with whom Mark and Sergio's teams were collaborating, T-cells that could recognise neoantigens from her tumour had been spotted.

All of this tied in with what was going on 'in real life' – Zarah's CT scan showed the tumour was stable in size, and her lymph nodes had the 'liquidy' appearance that had so baffled her clinical team at the time.

But then, suddenly, just after Cycle 6, with Zarah's chemo finished, the levels crashed back to zero, their activity suddenly silenced. What looked like a full-throated cytotoxic immune response, built up over months, seemed to have been snuffed out in a matter of weeks.

Separately, as part of his own PhD project, Pramit – Sophia's friend and colleague – had been looking at another aspect of Zarah's blood.

In particular, Pramit had been meticulously counting the number of rogue tumour cells floating in it, which is being studied as a possible marker of how active and aggressive a patient's disease is. This is an extremely tricky technique to perform, since tumour cells are rare in the blood and thus extremely difficult to fish out from the billions of other cells in a given sample. So – just as Sophia had been – Pramit had been using Zarah's blood samples to hone and perfect his skills.

In February, before she started chemotherapy, in every 10ml of Zarah's blood, Pramit found just three solitary floating tumour cells. But by August, after she'd finished chemo, the number had shot up sevenfold. This tied in with Sophia's observations – as the immune response was switched off, the cancer started to grow anew, shedding more and more cells into her blood supply.

What had happened? How had the tumour survived the chemotherapy and outwitted her immune system?

On a cold, dark, January evening, years later, I discussed all this data with Mark over a pint near UCL Cancer Institute. We considered a few possibilities, trying to build a theory of the case consistent with the data.

One possibility was that, under attack from the immune system, the cancer had acquired a new mutation, fuelling its growth but remaining invisible to the immune system.

Or, perhaps the damage from the chemo may have pushed the immune system ever harder to fight the cancer and the immune cells simply became exhausted, unable to stay on top of the rapidly growing cancer cells. Sophia's analysis had indeed revealed molecular signs of exhausted T-cells in Zarah's blood and urine.

But another suspect, Mark proposed, was a different group of immune cells – types of macrophage (see page 122 for a recap), known variously as tumour-associated macrophages, myeloid-derived suppressor cells, or M2 macrophages. Under normal circumstances, these are thought to be part of the late stages of wound healing, arriving at the end of the process, hoovering up damaged cells and resetting the activated cells back to a resting state. But in cancer terms, they're thought to be 'baddies' – invading into a tumour and shutting down the local immune response, allowing a tumour to grow free of attack. And while reading up on this, I'd spotted a research paper showing a curious thing:[3] it turns out that these suppressive macrophages are exquisitely sensitive to cisplatin chemotherapy – *the exact chemo drug that Zarah was being treated with.*

Unfortunately, Mark's team had not directly looked for these macrophages, so their involvement is no more than speculative. Nevertheless, here's what I propose happened – a slightly speculative, hand-wavy element of my theory of the case, but Mark's happy with it, and he's an expert.

Zarah's tumour was able to grow as it did because her initial immune response was held in check by invading macrophages, erroneously thinking they were helping heal a long-standing wound.

Then, when she started chemotherapy, the toxic drugs blitzed the cancer cells directly – releasing debris that stimulated local cytotoxic T-cells to try to break free of the macrophages' shackles. But the chemo also obliterated these macrophages themselves, and this, collectively, lifted the suppression of the T-cells in her tumour, setting them free to multiply in number and attack the tumour cells – bringing Zarah's cancer under temporary control.

On top of this, perhaps – as her chemo came to an end – one of the remaining tumour cells, as it divided catastrophically once more, acquired a new mutation, fuelling its growth. The immune system tired. The macrophages' number replenished. And so the T-cells' attack was, finally, snuffed out – and her tumour was able to start growing once more.

This may seem a little convoluted, but it's a completely reasonable extrapolation from Sophia's data, and also – more importantly – from what happened in real life. Soon after she stopped chemotherapy, Zarah's tumour returned with a vengeance.

On reading this, two obvious questions arise. Why stop taking cisplatin after just six cycles? And why use it in the first place if it seems so ineffective?

To answer the first question: cisplatin can cause serious damage to the rest of the body's systems – most notably the kidneys. Zarah put up with it pretty well, but many find it unspeakably tough. It's given in six cycles because clinical trials have shown that, on balance, this is the most effective dose – balancing out long-term side effects, while doing the maximum cancer killing.

But why use it at all? Primarily because – unlike the other chemo drugs we met in chapter 3 – in a small minority of people with bladder cancer, cisplatin has profound effects, and seems to be able to completely cure the disease. I remember Professor Peter Johnson – then Cancer Research UK's chief clinician (and now the NHS's clinical director for cancer) – telling me of a bladder-cancer-treating colleague who would occasionally remark, 'Bloody hell – chemo's cured another one.' Unfortunately, there's still no way to identify who will respond in this near miraculous way.

The second reason for using cisplatin is because, at the time Zarah was being treated, there wasn't really any alternative – aside, of course, from not having it, which is also a perfectly reasonable thing to do if, for whatever reason, you don't want to spend your remaining months regularly hooked up to a chemo pump and necking steroids to keep the nausea under control. As you have gathered, we felt differently, and knew the likelihood was that cisplatin would just buy us some time. Such are the awful choices with advanced cancer.

Since Zarah died, new options have begun to emerge, an unfolding story I've followed, as you can probably imagine, with a mixture of emotions. Immunotherapy is one. A new, sophisticated form of chemo, called enfortumab vedotin, is another. And a 'targeted' drug called erdafitinib is likely to arrive fairly swiftly too, for patients whose tumour carries a particular mutation. The bladder cancer oncologist's toolbox is now, finally, expanding. The challenge ahead will be to work out which patients will respond best to each one, and in what order or combination.

This will take years to unpick. So cisplatin – with all its upsides and downsides – will be around for a long time yet.

Sophia also made another, fascinating observation during her PhD – one that ended up in the pages of a scientific journal (and about which I wrote a heartfelt piece in the *Guardian* newspaper,[4] after discovering that Zarah's samples were involved). In separating out the T-cells from Zarah's urine, Sophia discovered that they bore a startling resemblance – in terms of the molecules on their surface – to the cells she was able to pluck out from her original tumour sample, even more so than the ones she spotted in Zarah's blood. This suggested that urine-derived T-cells could be used as an efficient way to monitor a patient's response to cancer treatment, without needing to take a biopsy. Such 'liquid' biopsies could prove incredibly useful in clinical trials.

After double-checking this phenomenon in more samples from other patients, and publishing the positive findings in a journal, Sophia's technique is now being employed in several cancer drug trials.

Not bad for an accidental PhD project. Zarah would be incredibly proud.

———

I want to step back slightly now and briefly discuss Zarah's lifelong urinary tract infections (UTIs) and whether they may have played a role in her cancer's development. It seems intuitive that they might have, but it's worth bearing in mind that about 20 per cent of women aged between 15 and 29 will develop a UTI, which will come back at least once in about 40 per cent of them. That's a *lot* of women. Conversely, the prevalence of bladder cancer in this age group is vanishingly small. If there's a link, it's a very, very weak one. But what does the evidence say?

In fact, the epidemiological evidence (and I suspect that I don't have to explain 'epidemiological' in our post-COVID world) cuts both ways. Some studies do, in fact, show a clear link. Others don't. Yet more – perhaps paradoxically – have even found a protective effect if someone regularly gets UTIs (perhaps, the authors propose, due to the enhanced anti-cancer immune activity in an infected bladder?).

Even among those who think the positive statistical link is real, there's debate about the nature of cause and effect, with critics pointing out that bladder tumours do, in fact, cause UTIs – a perfectly sensible argument, given what we've seen about how a growing tumour disrupts the normal integrity of the bladder's protective lining. But a review of the available evidence, published in 2016,[5] concluded:

'Inferences about the causal association between chronic urinary tract infections and bladder cancer risk should be drawn cautiously'

So, as far as this line of evidence goes, the jury is still out.

And yet.

I can't help but think back to a comment made to me by one of the researchers I spoke with for this book, Dr Jenny Rohn, a former cancer researcher who now studies UTIs. She pointed out that, in the normal bladder lining, the cells divide relatively slowly – a new cell is born every three to six months. This is slow compared with the lining of other bits of you: your gut lining, for instance, is replenished every few days.

Jenny also pointed out that when mice in the laboratory are given urinary tract infections (don't think too hard about how this is done), the resulting damage and inflammation causes bladder lining cells to divide much more rapidly – days, rather than weeks.

Which got me thinking.

Imagine a cell had already, by rogue accident, lost a key gene controlling its division – say, CDKN2A. As well as already being freed from normal control, the inflammation of a UTI might further accelerate its growth. Wouldn't this suggest that the accrual of new mutations – such as, say, the *TP53* gene – might happen sooner than otherwise?

So, no, I don't completely rule out Zarah's persistent UTIs having some sort of influence on whether – or, more specifically, *when* – she developed her tumour. Perhaps, in the spirit of Hanahan and Weinberg's Hallmarks model, it should be an 'enabling characteristic' rather than a cause *per se*. So, all things considered, I'm going to, tentatively, include it in the theory of the case. But only tentatively.

But! he said, metaphorically banging the desk. But! What is not in doubt, *at all*, is that, tragically, Zarah's history of UTIs – as with so many younger women with bladder cancer – meant that the symptoms of her cancer were overlooked, by everyone – herself, me, and her GPs – until it was too late to do anything about it.

The stats are clear: UTIs are more common in women. And women – particularly younger women – have a higher risk of dying from bladder cancer, because they're diagnosed later.

This is not a coincidence.

In June 2020, with the final draft of this book pretty much done and my publishers eager for me to submit, I received an email that I had almost given up hope of ever seeing.

'Dear Henry,' it began. 'This might be slightly late for your final draft but Zarah's samples are being sequenced this week and will be ready for analysis in 14 days. Best wishes, Chris'

Short, but to the point. It was, at last, the end of a long, stop-start, back-and-forth quest to find out what lurked in those samples – which had been taken at regular intervals throughout Zarah's treatment – and what it revealed about how her tumour had responded and adapted to chemotherapy, and when its growth had started accelerating. I was, simultaneously, massively relieved, slightly trepidatious about what my editor might say about yet another delay in submitting, and, as you might imagine, strangely nervous – even a bit fearful – about finding out what had been uncovered.

But before I get to the results, I should probably explain a bit about what exactly had been analysed, and how, and by whom.

As tumours grow and spread, the chaotic, disordered cells within them occasionally die and, as they do so, they release fragments of their contents into the bloodstream, including what's known as 'circulating tumour DNA', or ctDNA for short. Researchers have long suspected that measuring ctDNA in a patient's blood over time might allow their cancer's presence, or recurrence, to be monitored via a quick, non-invasive blood (or urine) test – a concept known widely as a 'liquid biopsy'. It's an elegant, simple idea, but turning it into a reality has been fraught with technical and scientific hurdles – chiefly the fact that, regardless of whether you have cancer or not, your blood contains traces of normal DNA from your normal cells, so to detect any tumour DNA you need a way to tell it apart from this background noise. It's needle-in-a-haystack stuff and was, for a long time, impossible to achieve with the sort of accuracy and speed needed to bring the idea from promising concept to clinical reality.

Over the past few years, however, huge leaps in both the cost and accuracy of DNA sequencing have moved liquid biopsies from concept to concrete. For a while, barely a month would pass without a hyped-up 'Simple Blood Test for Cancer' story appearing in the news, as competing groups around the world – often with commercial backing – sought to be the first to develop a reliable, useful, cost-effective liquid biopsy technique.

Among these groups, Charlie Swanton's team has been working on a particularly nuanced approach: to try to use the evolutionary 'trees' they generate from patients' tumours as a template from which to develop a sophisticated, highly personalised liquid biopsy test. Their idea is to first use multi-region sequencing to identify the characteristics of all the different clones in a patient's tumour. Then – using computer software and some very clever maths – for each clone, a subset of unique genetic faults is identified that can reliably identify ctDNA from each one, effectively generating a 'barcode' for every clone. This is used to make a suite of molecular probes, with which to effectively 'go fishing' in a patient's blood samples, looking for DNA fragments from each clone, and track how their levels change over time. In this way, a patient's unique tumour DNA provides a toolkit for its own monitoring – 'personalised medicine' at its most sophisticated.

In 2017, Charlie's team published their first attempt at this in the science journal *Nature*,[6] lending more weight to the idea that liquid biopsies could work in practice. Among a cohort of 100 patients with early-stage lung cancer, who'd all had surgery to remove their tumour, the team spotted several whose ctDNA levels started to rise suspiciously soon afterwards. These patients later had CT scans revealing that their tumours had indeed returned – as predicted by the ctDNA in their blood. It was a potential game changer: the ctDNA analysis picked up the returning tumours many weeks – and in some cases months – before they were large enough to be visible on a scan. The DNA fragments in the patients' blood also identified which of the clones from their original tumour were growing again, offering clues to potential treatments. As well as giving an early warning of their tumour's return, their analysis, and others like it, suggests that liquid biopsies could indeed offer doctors a means to modify a patient's treatment in a much more intelligent, personalised way. It was all very exploratory, lab-based research – no patients on the study actually had their treatment changed as a result, but it was an impressive proof of concept.

The lead author on that *Nature* paper was Chris Abbosh, a young, fresh-faced oncologist who works alongside Charlie at the Crick and UCLH. And it was Chris who'd sent me the email about Zarah's samples.

Chris has been busy since that 2017 finding, leading a project to scale up the meticulous, time-consuming laboratory processes they'd used in that research into something robust and rapid enough to be used in real time, in the NHS. A central partner in that project is a US-based company called ArcherDX, who are developing a particularly sensitive form of DNA analysis. Back in late 2019, upon learning that I'd hit a bit of an impasse with the plans for this book, Charlie Swanton had emailed Chris and a colleague at ArcherDX to ask if there was any way they could incorporate Zarah's samples in the next batch of lung cancer patients' samples they'd planned to analyse for Chris's project. They'd incredibly kindly agreed to do so, and so I'd put them in touch with Mark Linch at UCL to arrange for Zarah's blood samples to be shipped off to Denver, Colorado, frozen at -80°C.

But there the story – and the samples – had, frustratingly, got stuck. Quite understandably, since they were currently alive and being treated, the lung cancer patients' samples had to take priority. The team at Archer were still improving their methods, so things were moving slowly. It would likely take many months before Zarah's samples could be squeezed in. And then, of course, the COVID-19 pandemic arrived, and everything ground to a halt. I'd reluctantly accepted that my ambitions to have Zarah's samples analysed – and my search for answers – would have to be scaled back, if not abandoned entirely.

But then, just in time, Chris emailed. It was back on. The samples had been processed. The data were finally here.

Four weeks later – as befitting our newly adopted pandemic-era working practices – I joined Chris and Mark on a video call to discuss what they'd found in Zarah's blood, and what it revealed about how her tumour had evolved. Presenting the data was a young bioinformatician called Alex Frankell, who'd crunched the data from ArcherDX and linked it up with information on Zarah's treatments.

Pleasantries exchanged, Alex shared his screen. I held my breath.

What appeared was a graphical representation of tumour evolution called a fishplot. No acronyms involved – it just looks a bit like a fish. I've adapted it on the next page, and I'll try to explain what it represents.

FIGURE 4 How Zarah's tumour adapted to chemotherapy

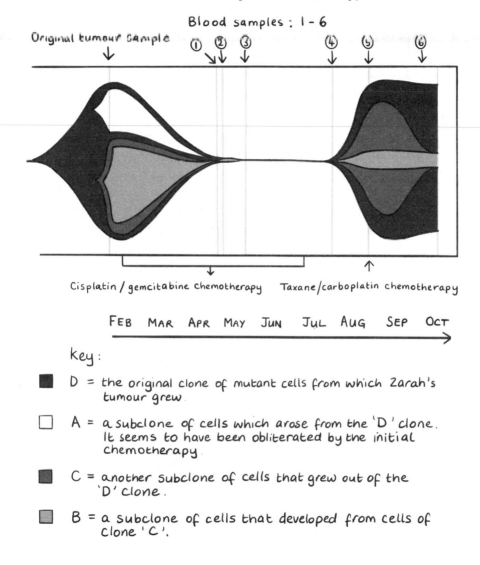

Blood samples : 1 - 6

Original tumour sample   ① ② ③   ④ ⑤   ⑥

Cisplatin / gemcitabine chemotherapy   Taxane/carboplatin chemotherapy

FEB MAR APR MAY JUN JUL AUG SEP OCT

key :

■ D = the original clone of mutant cells from which Zarah's tumour grew.

□ A = a subclone of cells which arose from the 'D' clone. It seems to have been obliterated by the initial chemotherapy.

■ C = another subclone of cells that grew out of the 'D' clone.

■ B = a subclone of cells that developed from cells of clone 'C'.

The line along the bottom – the x-axis – represents time, and as you follow the shaded blobs from left to right, you can see how the relative proportions of the different clones in Zarah's tumour rose and fell over time. Let's start on the left, and recap the initial data from the Crick. When she had her surgery and the original tissue sample was taken, the tumour had already evolved from its common ancestor (group D, in dark grey), which had spawned clones A (white) and C (mid-grey), the latter of which then spawned group B (pale grey). By this time, her tumour was mainly made of group B and group A cells, as depicted by the height of the two larger blobs.

Now follow the graph along, and look at what the blood samples reveal about what happened after her surgery, and during her initial cisplatin chemo. By mid-April – as we walked through the springtime woodland carpets of bluebells in the Chilterns, shocked, still coming to terms with Zarah's diagnosis – the first two samples contained relatively low levels of DNA, originating (and you'll have to look closely to see this) mainly from cells from 'mid-grey' group C and 'pale grey' group B.

By May, the next sample showed that the chemo seemed to have done a pretty good job… but not good enough. There were still traces of DNA present in her blood. The tumour – barely visible on the CT scan – was still very much alive.

Then, as we moved into a hot, balmy summer and Zarah continued, then completed, her chemo, things started to stir. By July – as her CT scan was showing that her disease was apparently 'stable'; as we holidayed in Barcelona; as we started discussions with Tom Powles about the possibility of an immunotherapy drug trial – sample 4 shows the cancer was already starting to return.

Then, over a 30-day period from late July to late August – as Zarah turned 38, and we joyfully got engaged – things started to snowball, rapidly: the ctDNA levels rose sharply. But again, look at the graphic. By the time sample 5 was taken, in late August, her tumour, now growing aggressively, was solely composed of cells originating from groups B, C and D. The palest 'A' cells had vanished entirely, apparently wiped out by the cisplatin chemo.

Now look at what happened next, at the effect of the last-ditch taxane chemotherapy she had in late August at Barts, as Tom tried valiantly to hold her disease in check while we waited for the trial to open. It did indeed have an effect – but only on the mid-grey, group C, cells. It had absolutely no impact on the cells descended from groups B (pale grey) and D (dark grey) – these continued their lethal growth, and by the time the final sample was taken, in mid-October, shortly before she died, the cancer spreading around her body was almost entirely made of cells that had arisen anew from that original type D clone.

After Alex had finished talking me through this data, with a few questions on the practicalities answered and grateful thanks offered, I pressed 'end call', and bit back a sob. What would have happened had we known any of this at the time? Could we have continued with the cisplatin? Pushed for an earlier switch to a new treatment? But which treatment? There was nothing else on offer, then, other than ineffective chemotherapy drugs, and there were no trials open at that time. As I said before, coulda, woulda, shoulda is a mug's game.

But, from a biological point of view, what does this add? How does this fit with our 'theory of the case'?

From one perspective, it doesn't really say anything new. We already know Zarah's tumour was affected by the cisplatin. We know it grew back rapidly. We know the harsh taxane chemo had little effect. We know – oh, how we know – that she died of cancer.

But think beyond Zarah's story for a minute, and think about the potential of this technique for people with cancer in future. As the data shows, it was apparent, from the blood samples taken around mid-June, that Zarah's cancer was growing again. But in 'real life', this was news we would only find out months later, in mid-August. Now think about the increasing number of promising new drugs in the pipeline, and how they're matched to particular mutations and hallmarks of cancer – which can, of course, be picked up by ctDNA analysis. As much as the data I've just shown you – this incredible deep-dive into the evolutionary dynamics of Zarah's tumour – change absolutely nothing about the past, just think about what they mean for the future: real-time, rapid analysis of how a person's cancer is responding to treatment, rather than waiting for a tumour to become visible on a CT scan, and the prospect of rapidly adapting treatment to try to contain the disease. Think how much more time this could buy people – even cure them. And, conversely, think how much unnecessary, harsh, gruelling treatment it could avoid.

We will get there, to this new, bright paradigm of cancer treatment. We will need to invest, heavily, in staff, training, time and research to get there, but we will. I'm sure of it.

There is one more, crucial piece of evidence I managed to track down to build my case, and map out What Happened In Zarah's Bladder: the results of the biopsy she had at Barts, in August 2016, as part of her enrolment on the BISCAY immunotherapy trial, led by Professor Tom Powles.

Aside from the biopsy's primary purpose – determining, based on the presence or absence of certain mutations, which 'arm' of the BISCAY study Zarah would be enrolled on to – I had long wondered what else the biopsy had uncovered. What other mutations had arisen over the course of her tumour's evolution? Were there any clues as to how it came back so aggressively?

Just like the ArcherDX blood analysis, tracking down this information took a lot of effort. Back in 2016, Zarah's biopsy sample had been sent over to AstraZeneca's facilities in the US, where DNA had been extracted and sent to another company, Foundation Medicine, for analysis. This threw up some fairly complicated bureaucratic and ethical hurdles. Despite me pestering Tom, and Tom pestering his contacts at AstraZeneca, nothing was forthcoming until after the initial findings of BISCAY had been released (we'll come to them later). Pharma companies, it seems, guard their secrets closely.

A PDF copy of Foundation Medicine's report finally dropped into my inbox one afternoon in late 2019 – several months before I was to receive the data from the blood samples. I was at work at the time so, naturally, I spent the afternoon ignoring my emails as I pored over it, googling the mutations it identified, silently trying to put the pieces together as my colleagues went about their work around me.

Here's what it contained, and what it implied.

Compared with the other analyses – by Charlie's team at the Crick, by Mark's group at UCL, and by ArcherDX – the Foundation Medicine report seemed almost shockingly lightweight. Rather than analysing the tumour cells' whole genomes, it had taken a more efficient approach, looking only at a subset of 395 genes (out of the 22,000 in the human genome), the rationale being that these genes have the strongest involvement in cancer, and, hence, they give the most useful information to a doctor trying to make clinical decisions for their patient. Which is entirely reasonable, if somewhat frustrating to me, after trawling through the incredible, macabre treasure trove of data I'd collated from the Crick and UCL (and, much later, from ArcherDX).

The report's findings were split into two sections, the first of which detailed well-understood mutations in cancer genes. In Zarah's sample, it listed seven gene aberrations.

The first two were familiar: the *TP53* R282W mutation, and the loss of *CDKN2A* – a validation of the Crick's findings, and reassurance that these two genes were absolutely fundamental players in Zarah's tumour.

The next three mutations listed, however, showed something new and unexpected. For a start, they all occurred in the same gene: *PIK3CA*, a gene that produces a protein intimately involved in regulating cell growth, and frequently found to be mutated in human cancers, and often associated with aggressive, fast-growing cancers (although relatively rare in bladder cancer).

All three mutations listed in the report were what is known as 'gain-of-function' mutations – in other words, they lead to the production of highly active, mutant forms of the protein, able to accelerate cell growth and multiplication.

It was also, I realised, ironclad evidence of a Darwinian phenomenon called 'parallel evolution' – nature's uncanny ability to come up with the same solution to a problem several times over. It's why so many species of animal use red as a warning signal, and why zebras, tigers and butterflies all use stripes to camouflage themselves. Nature always finds a way. Think back, for a moment, to the data from Zarah's blood samples I discussed earlier. At the time this biopsy was taken, the ctDNA data show that cells descended from three of the four clones in Zarah's tumour had found a way to grow back after the chemotherapy.

Three clones acquiring the ability to regrow; three separate growth-fuelling *PIKC3A* mutations.

Of course, there are other explanations, but as far as our 'theory of the case' goes, it's tempting to speculate that, taken together, these three separate *PIK3CA* mutations show that different clones in Zarah's tumour had all independently evolved the same solution to outmanoeuvre the pressures it was under – the chemotherapy's assault, and the immune system's attack. Darwinian evolution at work in its most devastating form.

And speculating further, this might have meant that Zarah's tumour would have been extremely sensitive to drugs that target mutant *PIK3CA* proteins. Such drugs exist, and existed back in 2016, but only in highly experimental forms on clinical trials. Like I say, coulda, shoulda, woulda: mug's game.

The rest of the report contained a few noteworthy nuggets. To learn more, I first shared it with a researcher in York, Dr Simon Baker, an expert in bladder cancer development, who spotted that two of the *PIK3CA* mutations bore the hallmarks of mutation by APOBEC proteins, suggesting that APOBECs were still ravaging Zarah's cancer's genome, even in the later stages of her disease.

I also looked into the two other genes in the main section of the report – *KDM6A*, which makes a protein that regulates gene activity, and *CDKN2B*, a 'sister' molecule of *CDKN2A*, similarly involved in controlling cell division. More evidence of the extreme chaos at play in the cells of the tumour as it spread.

I noted, with mild surprise, that the amplified *HER2* 'antenna' was missing from the report – likely due to the same issue Nicolai had spotted: it was amplified in too small a quantity to be spotted as abnormal. On the other hand, perhaps it was lost – in evolutionary terms – along the way, perhaps unnecessary given the development of the equally growth-enhancing PIK3CA mutations.

But without more information, all of this is more hand-waving speculation. Knowing that a gene is mutated in a tumour sample tells you little, on its own, about the effect of that mutation.

And the BISCAY trial?

Tom Powles presented its results at a large US cancer conference in 2019.[7] Frustratingly, it showed that while durvalumab immunotherapy was effective for some patients on the trial, adding the targeted drugs achieved little on top of this. It was, in essence, a negative trial.

But the real bittersweet kicker came a year later, when Tom presented the results of one of the other trials for which Zarah might have been eligible back in 2016, but which hadn't opened in time for her to enrol.

This time, there was no packed conference hall – COVID-19 had seen to that. So, over a video link, Tom shared data from a trial called JAVELIN-100, which had tested whether advanced bladder cancer patients would benefit from starting immunotherapy *as soon as they'd finished chemotherapy* – a 'maintenance' treatment, designed to put off their cancer's return for as long as possible.

It showed dramatic results – a big improvement in overall survival times, and a finding likely to change the way the disease is treated in future.[8] But too late for those who had the disease in the past. Too late for Zarah.

Such is science.

We've now finished our tour of the data I've been able to scrape together to tell this story, so let's recap everything we've learned over the last few pages, one last time.

Zarah's tumour arose from a cell in the upper right-hand side of her bladder, after it suffered catastrophic loss of a few vital genes – perhaps caused by 'friendly fire' from its own internal antiviral protection system, perhaps by tragic, random accident.

As it grew, slowly at first, but then faster – perhaps encouraged by the presence of persistent bacterial infections – it eventually doubled its genome and acquired the ability to fuel its own growth, kicking it into a higher gear. All this time, thanks to the continued action of rogue antivirus systems, it occasionally spawned new subclones bearing neoantigens, sending out weak signals to the immune system, which gently pruned it, weeding these odd mutant clones out, yet generally tending to ignore the majority of its growing bulk.

As the tumour continued to expand, the increasing rate of death in its disordered cells played a cruel trick, triggering a suppressive influx of wound-healing macrophages, slowing the immune-pruning and allowing the tumour cells to diversify into a number of different subclones, two of which became dominant. This expanding, variegated clump eventually grew so large it nearly filled her bladder, and – crucially – invaded through the muscle wall, and began to spread to her lymph nodes.

In January 2016, the advancing tumour finally made an error, revealing its presence to the wider world by blocking Zarah's urethra, causing her kidney to back up, and subjecting itself to harder, physical pruning – first by a surgeon's scalpel, and then by harsh chemotherapy drugs, obliterating many (but not all) of the remaining cells. But the chemo also destroyed the suppressive cells holding back her immune system, allowing it to attack the remaining cells. Together, this wiped out one of the dominant subclones that made up her tumour when she was diagnosed.

But, alas, a few cells survived unscathed – chemotherapy-resistant, hidden somehow from the immune system. From July, as levels of the chemotherapy dropped, and the immune suppression kicked back in, these cells – fuelled, perhaps, by newly acquired mutations – rapidly grew back, refilling her bladder, and spreading aggressively around Zarah's body.

By October 2016, the cancer cells were everywhere, consuming everything. They'd completely blocked her lymph nodes – causing catastrophic levels of fluid build-up around her body – and eroded her liver and lungs. Finally, they killed her.

I have only two further things to say in this chapter.

The first is about research on cancer, and the progress being made. I hope that this tale illustrates the awesome power of scientific research in revealing the disease's underlying biology – and yet also demonstrates how hard it is to convert this knowledge into ways to help people who develop it in the here and now. Collating the information in this chapter took years. As I know only too well, people with the disease often only have months. I once heard Charlie Swanton remark at a research conference, 'We're now able to learn much about a given patient's tumour that may improve our ability to treat it. Our challenge is to do so in a time frame that is clinically relevant for the patient.'

I am an optimist. I firmly believe that, one day relatively soon, analyses based on those described in this book – multi-region DNA sequencing, 'liquid biopsy' blood and urine analysis of tumour DNA, immune profiling and the rest – will be used in routine care, and completely transform cancer's treatment. But there are some big obstacles in the way – not least how we get the healthcare system back on its feet after the COVID-19 outbreak.

The second point I want to make is to hark back to a statistic I promised to reveal earlier in the book, in chapter 2.

Late one night, shortly after Zarah was diagnosed, while reading up online about bladder cancer – a form of the disease I then knew shockingly little about – I stumbled on a figure that caused me to draw breath: the average survival time for women affected with high-grade, stage 4 bladder cancer.

Women like Zarah.

I can no longer find the reference – it may be out of date by now. And at the time, I tucked it away in a corner of my brain, suppressed, to deal with at a later date. It was just a bit too shocking, back then. And after all, it was an average – there was no point in dwelling on it. But here it is:

Nine months.

Zarah was diagnosed on 23 January 2016. She died on 23 October that same year.

Exactly nine months.

It was, perhaps, the only average thing about her.

8

Some musings on cancer

To finish off, Jerry Springer-like, I want to leave you with some final thoughts, my reflections on cancer. This isn't, really, a manifesto for change, nor a neat, conclusory wrap-up with a series of punchy, clarion-like calls to action (although there may be the odd one or two). It's certainly not a guide to what to do, think, or feel if you yourself have cancer. It's barely even an ending. We've already, in a sense, had the ending.

Instead, it's more of a series of points I want to make – issues I want to get off my chest. Observations, if you will, on what I learned about a disease I thought I knew, then found out I didn't – but which I certainly do now. Some of what follows might get a bit soapboxy. Other bits are merely some musings on a variety of topics between which I joined unexpected dots – the little 'aha!' moments that occurred from time to time. Some of it may, indeed, be mere wittering.

But regardless, I hope some of it is useful and, perhaps, thought-provoking. If you've had cancer, or – like me – had a close personal brush with it, some of it will doubtless be familiar. I hope it resonates. If you're in the medical or scientific sphere, I hope some of this doesn't come across as too finger-waggy or naive. If you're a policymaker or research funder, I hope some of it gives you pause to consider how you might help effect change (or encouragement that your current direction of travel is, at least, forward).

And if – like so many people for most of their lives – cancer is something that has yet to inveigle its way in, in the awful way it can, then I hope it gives you an insight into what, for so many of us, is a reality, an ordeal, a passion, a profession, or an obsession.

Right, OK, that's enough mildly apologetic preamble. Let's get into it, one last time.

———

I want to start off by talking about the NHS.

The 2020 outbreak of a pandemic coronavirus, SARS-CoV-2, has brought the UK's healthcare system to the forefront of public life, with healthcare workers applauded weekly, by almost the entire British public. NHS staff have dealt with the crisis heroically, and this has rightly been recognised.

But similarly, the pandemic has highlighted the chronic lack of resources we've made available to our healthcare system over the last decade – even as record amounts are pumped into it, to prop it up in the white heat of a national crisis.

There was a period in our recent history when UK government ministers were rather fond of saying that we could only afford to fund the healthcare system if the economy were 'properly' managed. The unprecedented economic damage wrought by COVID-19 has flipped that causality around. We simply must fund the NHS properly.

So, yes, cards on the table: I am a huge fan of the NHS. The idea of a single nationwide healthcare system, that doesn't link your coverage to your employment status, that's available throughout your life without needing to pay extra for certain treatments, is a beautiful thing – and we should be proud to live in a country where this basic concept is still, broadly, unchallenged. And it's more than an idea – in practical terms, the NHS is a service that helps thousands of people every day, and is full of the most incredible, dedicated, hard-working staff. Long live the NHS, and all who sail in her.

Of course, it is not perfect, but many amazing people dedicate their careers to making the NHS constantly better – both the 'front line' staff and the hundreds who work behind the scenes to make it all tick. They do vitally important things – not least, reacting with admirable speed when pandemics hit, to make sure as many people with cancer as possible can be treated safely – and I love them for it. This little ramble is no slight on them.

But I want to dwell for a moment on Zarah's experience of the NHS – four years before the coronavirus outbreak – and what it taught me about the practical, day-to-day effects of its systemic lack of funding.

Perhaps one of the most important things I learned – something that may seem profoundly obvious to some – is the difference between 'treatment' and 'care'.

When you see a doctor, what you usually want is treatment. But what you actually receive – or should receive – is something extra: care.

I've come to realise that 'care' is the treatment itself, plus a load of unseen, ancillary 'stuff' that, if done well, should be almost unnoticeable. The seamless booking of a follow-up appointment. The letter to your GP. The entry of information into a database. The smile. The sympathy. The chit-chat. The porter who takes you from the ward to your scan. The cleaner who empties the bin in the corner of surgery. The remembering of your name.

This may seem a profoundly obvious point, but it struck me at several points during Zarah's illness that, when things became stressful and frustrating, and too much to bear, quite often what was going on was that something in that broad, nebulous cloud of 'care' wasn't quite lined up. Zarah received, in the main, quite exemplary treatment. But on a few (thankfully rare) occasions, as you'll have seen over the course of this book, the care she had was lacking.

A consequence of poor care, it seems to me, is that as well as feeling a bit crappy, or ignored, or angry, or rushed, the patient (or their carer) has to devote time and energy into managing these things themselves – calling to check appointments, trying to find a nurse, explaining the situation to yet another doctor, trying to get answers as to why things were taking so long.

In one way, you can regard 'treatment' as a mere protocol – a series of steps to be followed to make a patient better. But care – as I'm defining it (and it's my book, I'll define it how I want to, thank you very much) – is the collection of essentially human kindnesses that surround these steps. To illustrate, an example: the quite different experiences Zarah had on two adjacent wards on the same floor of the same hospital can only really be explained in terms of people, and of human interactions. The treatment was the same, but the care was different. That's not to say that the staff on one ward were intrinsically 'nicer' people than on the other, more that the way they interacted – both with each other, and with Zarah, and with me – led to an emergent property, greater than the sum of its parts, that was superior in one ward to the other: better care.

What lies at the heart of this? Probably loads of different factors, and I'm sure there's a sizeable body of academic work looking at how to break them down, measure them and improve them. But it struck me that a fundamental component of good quality care is, quite simply: time.

Time to prepare for an appointment. Time for professional and patient to understand one another. Time to frame bad news. Time to understand what's been discussed. Time to think. Time to ask questions. Time to write notes. If I were the sort to invent simplistic pseudo-scientific equations to try to explain complex social phenomena, I might be tempted to go with something like: $CARE = TREATMENT \times TIME$.

As I write this, the UK healthcare system – our beloved NHS – is in something of a pickle. It is staffed with wonderful, knowledgeable people who work their bloody socks off – but is seriously underfunded and understaffed. And while the stats on treatment outcomes seem to be, broadly, holding up (if anything, cancer survival is actually slowly increasing), this is only because its staff are working incredibly hard, round the clock, to hold the thing together. But unfortunately, it seems that the quality of care people feel they receive is suffering. Over the last few years, the British Social Attitudes survey has revealed a declining public satisfaction with the NHS, dropping, in 2018,[1] to a low not seen since 2007.* There are, of course, broader socio-political issues at play here, not least the way the NHS has been used as a political punchbag by a series of fairly low-powered politicians and commentators. But it's hard to convince oneself that there isn't a real phenomenon underpinning the drop-off. (It must be noted, however, that within this broader trend, satisfaction with NHS cancer services, as measured by the annual National Cancer Patient Experience Survey, has broadly held up,[2] despite growing waiting times – a testament to both the political priority given to cancer, and the efforts of the staff who treat and manage it).

---

*The latest report, in 2019,[3] showed a partial reverse in this decline, which the report's authors attribute to the announcement, shortly before the survey was carried out, of extra funding for the NHS.

Here's another statistic – linked to the previous one – that paints a depressing figure: largely due to demographics (i.e. more older folks), the number of people treated in hospitals* each year has increased by 21 per cent over the last decade.[4] But over the same period, real-terms NHS funding in England has increased by just 14 per cent[5] – nowhere near sufficient to keep up with the increase in demand. Can you imagine any commercial entity – say, a widget manufacturer – responding to a 20 per cent increase in demand with a mere 14 per cent increase in resources? It's madness. Absolute, unsustainable madness. But here's my point: in a healthcare system, delivering treatment effectively and safely is absolutely paramount. And if the same number of staff have to treat a rapidly increasing number of patients with only slightly more resources, they have an ever-diminishing amount of time to devote to all the other little things. And so, to balance that equation I certainly didn't make up just now, and *definitely* am not about to then use to make a point (oh, OK then), you could argue that the first thing to suffer when healthcare resources get tight is time. And as I've argued above, when time is in short supply in a healthcare system, and the number of people treated (safely and properly) increases, it's the surrounding care that suffers.

And so, when I now look at the ongoing debate over healthcare funding, about billion-pound budgets, and X per cent increases in this or that spending, or the spiralling costs of new cutting-edge treatments – I can't help thinking that, if the goal is not just to improve treatment but to improve people's care, we've got the units wrong.

We shouldn't be thinking in terms of money. We should be thinking about pumping more *time* into the system.

Of course, to invoke another made-up equation, TIME = MONEY, and you can't, say, hire more staff without big wodges of cash. Nor can you magically make being a doctor or nurse an attractive, less stressful, sustainable job. The NHS, in fact, has a huge number of unfilled roles across the board, from nursing to endoscopy. What, you might ask, is preventing these roles from being filled?

---

*as measured by 'finished consultant episodes', defined as: 'time a patient spends in the continuous care of one consultant using the hospital site or care home bed(s) of one health care provider (or, in the case of shared care, in the care of two or more consultants)'.

So it strikes me that the public debate about the NHS is so often framed in terms of cash being 'something that's spent on treatments' (particularly drugs), rather than something that buys time for **care**, and to make a job more attractive. And I wonder what might happen if the discourse around NHS funding were to shift to something that talked more about time and care, rather than money and drugs.

Aside from time, there's another aspect of care I want to dwell on – and I am most certainly not the first to raise it: integration vs fragmentation.

Until Zarah got cancer, I had never realised quite how many moving parts there were in the NHS that had to – in some way – cooperate and communicate with each other to keep the show on the road. NHS England, Cancer Alliances, STPs, Trusts, CCGs, GPs, private providers, social enterprises, social care services, hospices, charities – all of these different organisations or groups, and more, make up the environment through which people with cancer must travel. And that's before we get to the different departments and specialisms within an individual hospital – oncology, radiology, urology, cardiology, pathology, pharmacy and the like.

When things work as intended – like the proverbial swan, paddling furiously yet moving serenely – you don't, as a patient or carer, notice the effort involved in coordinating it all. You just get good care, and so you can focus on getting through your treatment. And I do want to emphasise the fact that Zarah received some fantastic care during her illness.

But when things don't go so well – when the gaps appear, and you fall down them… my word, it gets confusing, and frustrating, and overwhelming. And it doesn't half affect the experience of the care you receive.

Now, as I said, I'm not the first to make this point – the idea of 'integrated healthcare' is top of the contemporary lexicon of healthcare policy-wonkery. But so much of what I see as the current direction of travel – certainly in the macro-scale sense – seems to be in the opposite direction. From former prime minister David Cameron's broken promise of 'no more top-down reorganisation of the NHS', to his predecessor Tony Blair's introduction of market-based reforms – it's all led to a confused and confusing structure, which, from a patient perspective, can be a nightmare to navigate.

There are noble efforts underway to ameliorate this, including – across England – new organisations called 'Integrated Care Systems', or ICSs, which aim to defragment the system by bringing NHS organisations, local councils and others together to coordinate and share resources. And I certainly don't want to get into the whole debate about privatisation. However, there is of course a paradox, because not all fragmentation is necessarily 'bad'. The NHS's critics point out, with much justification, that a large, centralised, bureaucratic healthcare system can be its own worst enemy. Decisions tend to be made on a national level, and handed down to local systems, sometimes with little consideration for 'on the ground' matters. The 2010 NHS reforms were driven, in part, by a laudable desire to hand back control to local collectives of GPs – so-called clinical commissioning groups – to try to make the system more responsive and more 'patient-centred'.

So perhaps the real questions – applicable to all healthcare systems – are these: how do you best balance centralisation vs localisation? How do you reap the benefits of both? How do you design a system that offers consistent standards, for all patients, while allowing local systems to adapt to the particular needs of people in that particular area? Perhaps the real discussion should be one freed of the ideological baggage around private v state-owned, insurance v single-payer, and all the rest: how do we find a model that yields the highest possible levels of satisfaction, and good health, among people who use it?

So if I were to have five minutes to rant at a senior politician about what he or she should do about the NHS, my message would be this: stop being so bloody careless with your healthcare reforms.

And let's not ignore the funding elephant any longer. For any reforms to be successful, a system needs resources to adapt. So give the NHS some more bloody money, for some more staff, so the badly overworked ones that already dedicate their lives to helping people have more time to do so.

The second topic I want to dwell on is clinical research in general, and clinical trials for people with advanced cancer in particular.

As you'll have seen from our story, being able to enrol on a trial was an incredible source of hope, both for Zarah and for me – a chink of light in the gloom, a door through which we might walk to some sort of future. Part of this, of course, was the nature of the drugs we were hoping to get access to – the checkpoint immunotherapies that can, for some, produce dramatic results (although as Annabell's story illustrates, even when they 'work', the long-term effects can be incredibly tough to bear).

Clinical trials, of course, have far wider benefits than to their participants – they're the lifeblood of medical research, the tried-and-trusted way to keep medicine moving forward, to discover new treatments, to refine their use, to minimise harms, and – just as importantly – to find out what *doesn't* work.

Because not every experimental therapy available in trials will be as promising as checkpoint immunotherapy. And when it comes to early phase studies – the very first-in-human, super-experimental stuff – about 9 out of 10 people, in fact, don't benefit directly from the treatment under study.[6] The history of medical progress is littered with good ideas that never panned out.

And yet, thanks to studies both positive and negative – and the heroic people who run them, and take part in them – medicine continues to advance, and disease becomes ever more conquerable. Just consider the incredible global effort now underway to tackle the COVID-19 coronavirus.

But just to focus on evidence and progress, and altruism and all that, is to miss a fundamental point about what trials can represent on an individual level: a profound source of hope. When you're slogging your way through seemingly endless rounds of chemotherapy, or facing the prospect that the last approved therapy might not work for you, or crossing your fingers while waiting for your next scan result, the knowledge that there's a trial available – that there's something new that might just help – can make the difference between being able to get out of bed or not, to inject yourself in the stomach with anticoagulant, to struggle up and down the stairs in pain because the physio said it was the best thing for you, even though every fibre of your body wants to just curl up and cry. Clinical trials are hope, distilled into medical practice. Hope that keeps you gritting your teeth through the dark times. And with cancer, there are always dark times.

So as the powers-that-be try to improve the UK's overstretched healthcare system, as well as making sure there's time to care, there needs to be just as much effort to make sure that doctors have time to do research – to think about it, plan it, and carry it out – and to discuss it with their patients.

There are benefits to this beyond the obvious. It boosts morale: staff involved in research are more engaged with their work. And it boosts outcomes: patients at research-active clinical centres do better – even those who aren't on research studies – because these centres attract the best minds and most cutting-edge treatments.

The building blocks for all this are already there. The UK is fortunate to have a thriving medical research community, and at any one time there are about 2000-odd clinical trials open to patients around the country, including around 600 for people with cancer[7] (at least, there were until the bloody coronavirus forced many to be paused – at least, we hope, temporarily).

In the UK, about 20 per cent of patients take part in trials[8] – one of the highest statistics anywhere in the world. This is an extraordinary thing – as extraordinary as the NHS – and something we should similarly cherish and protect. And yet, just as with the NHS, we could be doing even better. Too few people say they have conversations with their doctors about research. The most recent National Cancer Patient Experience Survey – a regular barometer of how people with cancer feel about their care[9] – found that only a third of patients report that they've spoken with their care team about the prospect of taking part in research, a figure that's remained more or less in the same ballpark for a considerable period.

There are, of course, all sorts of barriers in the way to moving this statistic upwards, offering more hope to more people with cancer (although giving doctors more time to have these conversations would be a start).

Trials can have strict entry criteria, and even with 600 trials open, there are, at any one point in time, nearly three million people with cancer in the UK, with around 370,000 more diagnosed every year. But according to the National Institute of Health Research, only around 67,000 of them took part in some form of cancer research study last year.[10] That's a lot of people with cancer who don't take part in research, and a huge shortfall in capacity should everyone wish to do so.

So despite much lofty rhetoric about 'a trial for every patient', there's a very long way to go to make this a reality.

But at risk of a slightly circular argument, that's not to suggest that the simple answer is just to open thousands more trials. Clinical research needs to be rigorous and hypothesis driven. The NHS has a simplistic, well-meaning goal of getting more people on to trials – but this runs the risk of incentivising poor-quality medical research. There is always a balance to be struck – and, paradoxically, it's very likely to shift further away from 'opportunity for all'. A trend towards more 'stratified' medicine, where patients are recruited because they fit criteria defined by sophisticated molecular tests, means that trials are becoming smaller and more targeted. Opportunities are becoming scarcer, simply because scientists are getting better at clinical research.

But these complexities aside, there's another reason why 'more trials' is an over-simplistic solution. It's that, even when they're up and running, trials can struggle to recruit, and some never even manage to recruit enough patients to meet their objectives – a tragic loss of time and money.

Again, there are some valid reasons for this – but in the case of advanced cancer trials, one is quite simple: some people die before they have a chance to enrol.

So, I have an idea.

To illustrate it, consider this. Zarah was fortunate enough to live in London, and be treated at some of the best research-active medical centres in the world. And yet it was only when she'd finished her initial chemotherapy that she was transferred over from UCLH to Barts, and conversations began about immunotherapy trials. Even when this had started, there were still a few issues in transferring her care over from one NHS Trust to another.

And even more, once there was a suitable trial open for her, there was still a long delay before she was able to receive durvalumab immunotherapy (a delay that – we now know, thanks to Tom Powles' JAVELIN trial – may have substantially shortened her life). And the key reason for the delay was the long and drawn-out process of getting the data together – particularly the blood test results – to prove that she met the trial's entrance criteria. This was despite the fact that, in the preceding months and weeks, she'd had multiple appointments, during which a large volume of routine information was collected about her. For reasons I've never properly understood, none of this information seemed to count towards the trial enrolment – she needed to provide a 'fresh' set of results specifically for the trial.

This whole process, of course, took time – and during that time, her condition deteriorated. When someone is facing a fast-moving, rapidly evolving cancer, every day counts.

So every blood sample, every assessment, every interaction with the NHS should count too.

So here's a thing. Why don't we consider, as we've come to do with organ donation, some sort of presumption of 'opt-in' for medical research for progressive incurable conditions, so that as people's disease inevitably advances, their data is continually collected and recorded and available to triallists, to speed up the enrolment process?

I'm not, for a minute, suggesting that the essential processes of consent and ethics are compromised. But there must be a way for clever people to get their heads together and find ways to speed up this process, and make sure everyone with advanced cancer, who wants to, has a chance to benefit from experimental cancer therapies – and a chance to have their data used to help others after they're gone.

Now, I've been describing medical research as if it were exclusively concerned with developing new treatments – in particular, testing new drugs in clinical trials. That, of course, is only a partial picture. Medical research involves a broad range of different disciplines, from finding ever more ingenious ways to unpick the inner workings of the human body (a field often called 'basic' or 'discovery' research), to understanding the psychological impact of different conditions on people (psychosocial research), and the tracking of patterns of diseases in society (epidemiology) – and much more in between. (And of course, there's more to clinical trials than drugs – they can test any medical intervention: surgical techniques, types of radiotherapy, different ways of diagnosing or monitoring a disease – etc.)

All of it is incredibly important, every field part of a giant web of interconnected, ever-expanding knowledge of how to improve human health. But (perhaps because it's less obviously and immediately beneficial to people with disease) not all of it gets the same attention as do clinical trials.

So I now want to share a few thoughts on what might be broadly described as the 'research agenda', particularly on a few aspects of it that are (even) more important to me now than they were at the beginning of this story.

First, a burgeoning field often known as 'translational' research.

There has, historically, been a perception of a clear dividing line in the medical research community. On the one side of it, you have the laboratory scientists – biologists, biochemists and others – whose stereotypical habitat is the laboratory, whose garment of choice is the lab coat, and whose preferred state of being is hunched over some sort of complex instrument: a microscope, say, or a spectrometer or a tissue culture unit (or, increasingly, a laptop); peering, detachedly, into biology's deepest mysteries.

On the other side, you have the clinical researchers — often jobbing doctors with an interest, and training, in research methods, motivated by the prospect of improving things for the people they see every day, their patients.

Like all stereotypes, there is more than a grain of truth to it. But it is also a very blurry line, if it really exists at all. In the late 1980s, I was in my teens, approaching my A-levels and wondering what to do next – medicine or biochemistry. I did some work experience at my local hospital: St George's, in Tooting, South London. Over a period of months, I shadowed a young medic who, as part of his training, was doing a PhD in cardiovascular research. On some days, I'd sit with him in his clinic while he saw his desperately unfit, wheezy, sweaty patients; on others, we'd spend long hours in the tissue culture laboratory, where he'd teach me how to grow cells in a Petri dish, and then carry out experiments on them to understand how they grew. (Callous teenager that I was, I didn't care for the patient stuff, so off I went to study biochemistry.)

So there's always been a somewhat fuzzy line dividing those at the laboratory bench and those at the patient's bedside. And yet the division of labour has often been fairly simple, the flow of information across it unidirectional: the laboratory researchers make their observations, then the clinical researchers dream up ways to put them to use to benefit patients.

But in recent years, partly driven by the advent of a whole slew of sophisticated new research techniques – not least the ability to sequence a human genome in rapid time – these two disciplines have moved into ever closer proximity, their aims and priorities ever more closely aligned. Research institutes have arisen within or immediately proximate to hospitals. It's not uncommon, in some cases, for laboratories to be literally down the corridor from a ward.

With this mutually constructive orbit, the further blurring of the line, have come deeper and more relevant insights into how diseases develop, evolve and respond to treatment. Petri dishes, plastic tubes and lab animals will always have their place, but as well as scrutinising archived blocks of frozen tissue, or decades-old, immortal cell lines, researchers are now, increasingly, being employed to study fresh samples taken directly from a patient being currently treated. And as a result, new insights tumble apace out of the lab, down the corridor, and into the clinic.

As an example, consider Sophia's research paper, which I mentioned in the previous chapter, and which was published two years after Zarah's death. This, you may remember, was an analysis of immune cells in the urine of bladder cancer patients – Zarah among them – and the discovery that these cells appear to have come from within the tumour, and thus bear clues as to the nature of the molecular hide-and-seek being waged between it and the immune system. This discovery raises the potential that whether, and how, a patient is responding to treatment might be monitored via a quick urine test, rather than by repeatedly, invasively, taking tissue from their bladder. The researchers at UCL and elsewhere are now, as I write this, incorporating this concept into various ongoing trials, to test their theory. It's a wonderful example, I feel, of what's meant by translational research – samples from a patient are studied in a lab, observations noted and interpreted alongside their clinical data, predictions made, and later incorporated into new clinical studies to find out if they're useful.

Similarly, the inroads that teams like Charlie Swanton's are making into understanding cancer evolution, and the heterogeneity of cells within a tumour, are only possible because of the patients who consented to have their biopsies and bodily fluids analysed by the Crick's powerful DNA sequencers.

And so, when I talked earlier about 'taking part in research', I didn't just mean enrolling on a trial. I meant that, as patients make their uncertain journey through the health system, we need to get better at making sure that as much value as possible is gleaned from every data point, every biopsy, every blood sample, every questionnaire that they generate on the way – and that this information is used to improve the lives of those who will, later, inevitably, walk that same path.

This is not trivial. After Sophia's paper was published, and I wrote about this issue in a national newspaper, I was contacted by a variety of (broadly sympathetic) experts, who helpfully pointed out some of the barriers that stand in the way. Samples and data must be used in rigorous research studies, not sitting idly in freezers 'just in case'. Data protection, consent, funding, ethics – and, of course, time – all matter.

But, come on, let's just dream for a moment. How extra-amazing would the NHS be if it were, in itself, a giant networked clinical research platform, with all patients' data and outcomes collected, then carefully scrutinised for clues as to how to treat others? How much more rapid the progress?

We should dare to have that dream.

But even if this fantasy did become a reality, true progress will only come if researchers are asking the right questions of the data, and yield answers that are genuinely transformational. Zarah's experience – particularly those occasions where, in answer to persistent questioning, the answer still came back as 'we don't really know' – made me wonder if, perhaps, there are a few questions that aren't getting as much attention as they should. Certainly, these are the areas that, along with rigorous translational research, I now regard as personally important.

So here are a few ideas for research questions that, perhaps, could get a bit more prioritisation from medical research funders.

From its very inception, the vast majority of research into cancer has focused on one outcome above all: improving survival for people affected by it. Finding ways to extend their lives, if not cure them outright.

It's been a long slog, but we can now look back on some incredible progress. To quote from Cancer Research UK's own analysis, in the 1970s only around a quarter of people with cancer in the UK survived for 10 years or more. By the 2010s, that proportion had risen to half.[11] Half! When you consider everything I've written about cancer in this book – its malleable, Darwinian capacity to evolve and adapt; the incredible range of biological tricks it can pull out of the bag to evade treatment – the fact that medical science has given us the ability to keep this once uniformly lethal disease at bay, or cure it, in half of all people who get it, is nothing short of remarkable. And this is from an analysis done just before the advent of the next generation of treatments – immunotherapies, targeted therapies and the rest. So it seems likely that this hopeful trend will continue upwards.

So perhaps it's time to start shifting some resources – not all, but much more than currently – towards finding better ways to manage the disease's effects, as well as trying to cure it.

Macmillan Cancer Support estimates that there are about three million people in the UK who are living with, or beyond, a diagnosis of cancer.[12] As the population ages, and more people get cancer as a result, a figure that's predicted to rise to four million by 2030 – a staggering number. These include people who suffered like Annabell did – people who've lost their hearing, or have arthritis, or chronic fatigue, or pain. They deserve answers to the ills that ail them while they live with their cancer, whatever the eventual outcome.

What, for instance, is the underlying biology of lymphoedema? How can we prevent it? What's the best way to treat it? Can it be reversed? Are diuretics better than lymphatic drainage?

Can we develop, for people with chronic pain, some sort of high-strength painkiller that doesn't cause painful constipation, nor put them into a soporific, zombie-like state? (This latter point would be amazing even for people with incurable cancer: there were so many things I'd like to have said to Zarah – and for her to hear them – towards the end.)

Is there a way to track and monitor recurrent, persistent infections – the sort that people going through treatment for cancer pick up regularly throughout their treatment – in real time, rather than having to wait for bugs to grow in a Petri dish far away from the ward?

And can we find better, more sophisticated ways to track and monitor cancer itself, so that fewer people have to hear the uncertain words, 'Well, we *think* your scan looks OK'?

There are research groups, of course, working on all of these questions – but often in the margins, in relative isolation, and certainly not with the incredible financial resources bestowed upon those who quite justifiably seek to extend life, but without necessarily improving it.

As survival rates drift ever upwards, I can't help but think it's time for... if not a rethink, then a serious taking of stock.

On the topic of prioritisation, and profile, I want to talk about bladder cancer itself. Because since Zarah died I've come to learn quite a lot about the disease.

And what I've discovered paints a fairly depressing picture.

Over my years working at Cancer Research UK – particularly since social media became a 'thing' – I've always been intrigued by a particular phenomenon. Whenever we communicate to the public the results of a research on a particular cancer type, we almost always get comments that can broadly summed up as: 'That's all very well, but what about *my* type of cancer?' We then have to draft a slightly defensive response, most usually explaining that we do indeed fund research on that type of cancer, and also a whole boatload of basic, fundamental research that's led to insights relevant to all forms of cancer.

The overall phenomenon – what about me? – can, in a remote, detached, professional way, be quite irritating, especially when you've spent hours carefully drafting text explaining and contextualising some intricate scientific discovery. Partly, I guess, that's an inevitable result of working for a large national organisation that funds research into a disease that has so many different types – you can't speak to everyone at once. But still, our responses, despite their cheerful, sympathetic tone, are occasionally typed with slightly irked fingers.

But I'm now going to be 'that guy', and advocate for a greater focus on bladder cancer. Because, since Zarah's death, with everything I've since learned, I've come to what I think is the justifiable view that bladder cancer research is indeed an under-studied, under-resourced, under-networked field – and that bladder cancer itself is a disease that deserves quite a bit more public and professional attention. Let me explain why.

As I've worked, over the years, on a variety of stories and projects, I've become pretty familiar with the lie of the land, so to speak, with a range of different types of cancer – so much so that I've come to carry with me, in my head, a sort of dark version of the game 'Top Trumps' – a top-line summary of the unique features of different forms of the disease. So, if you say to me 'prostate cancer', I'll immediately be thinking of a relatively common disease, chiefly of older men who find they need to go to the loo a lot, or not at all; one that's linked to testosterone, can be diagnosed (imperfectly) with the PSA blood test, and which has slow-growing and fast-growing forms. The phrase 'brain tumour' causes me to think of a constellation of 200 different diseases with weird names like 'astrocytoma', and 'diffuse intrinsic pontine glioma', the causes of which are relatively opaque, has something to do with stem cells, and for which the prognosis is often bleak. 'Bowel cancer' – most cases linked to diet, others to a host of known inherited risk factors, increasing rates in younger people, screening programme, curable if caught early. 'Ovarian cancer' – vague symptoms, difficult to diagnose, few known causes, often very sensitive to platinum chemotherapy, can keep coming back. For each, I could probably even give you a rough ballpark figure for how many people are diagnosed each year, and, possibly, a few interesting scientific discoveries in the field.

But when Zarah was first diagnosed with bladder cancer, I drew a blank. I had some vague sense that it had once been linked to old-fashioned, long-disused hair dyes, but beyond that, my oncological Top Trump card was devoid of detail. I could remember working on, perhaps, a couple of stories on the subject: I visited the news archive on the Cancer Research UK website, and filtered the content by cancer type. Since 2003, the charity has published fewer than 50 items tagged with 'bladder cancer', compared with nearly 700 on breast cancer, 300-odd for each of lung and bowel cancers, and 240 for prostate cancer.

Maybe, I thought, it was relatively rare. So I went and looked at the statistics on the Cancer Research UK website. Here are the rounded number of cases diagnosed, for the most common 14 types of cancer, in 2016:

1) Breast cancer	55,000
2) Prostate cancer	48,000
3) Lung cancer	47,000
4) Bowel cancer	42,000
5) Melanoma	16,000
6) Non-Hodgkin lymphoma	14,000
7) Kidney cancer	13,000
8) Head and neck cancers	12,000
9) Brain tumours	11,000
10) Bladder cancer	**10,000**
11) Pancreatic cancer	10,000
12) Womb cancer	9500
13) Leukaemias	9500
14) Oesophageal cancer	9000

Bladder cancer is the tenth most common cancer. What did I make of that? OK, it was a bit odd that I knew basically nothing about it, but I wasn't, you know, shocked and appalled. I put my lack of awareness down to my own ignorance as much as any wider issue... and then events overtook – I didn't really think much more about the bigger picture until afterwards.

But after Zarah died, particularly after I was invited to take up a role as a patient advocate on a national bladder and kidney cancer research committee, I began to think about bladder cancer a lot more. About why there was so little public discussion about it. About why it was treated the way it was. About why so few researchers took an interest in it. And, in the process, I learned about a rather different form of the disease to the one Zarah had – a form called 'non-muscle invasive' bladder cancer – a good number of which, for reasons we'll come to shortly, aren't included in the stats I've just listed.

Like muscle-invasive bladder cancer (the form Zarah had), 'non-muscle invasive' cancer starts in the lining of the bladder. But, as the name suggests, these tumours haven't yet invaded into the muscle that surrounds the bladder – a tissue rich in blood vessels and lymphatic vessels, which provide the cancer cells a means by which they can escape throughout the body. These non-muscle invasive tumours can be removed from the bladder with surgery, and for many, this is the end of the story – an operation to remove a growth, a brush with cancer (their doctor might not have even used the word 'cancer'), and on with normal life.

But for a substantial proportion of people with this form,* the disease keeps coming back. Again. And again. For the rest of their lives. They will need regular monitoring – i.e., a camera up the pee-hole – forever. And when it does come back, the treatment involves a stay in hospital for an operation just like the one Zarah had in Westmoreland Hospital – a transurethral resection, or TURBT, under general anaesthetic, to remove and analyse the tumours. In patients whose disease looks, or becomes,

---

* Estimates vary, but a paper published in 2009 estimated that, after 5 years, between 30 and 80 per cent of people with a non-muscle invasive cancer will have had a recurrence.[13]

particularly abnormal, they can also have a rather crude treatment whereby they have a dose of the bacteria that makes up the BCG vaccine (yes, that one – the one you probably had at school, to give you lifelong protection against tuberculosis) squirted into their bladder, and then have to roll around on a bed to ensure it coats the whole of the inside surface. And then for several days, they usually have flu-like chills and shivers, and a nasty burning sensation when they pee. It's a bizarre treatment, developed in the 1970s, which appears to work as a particularly crude immunotherapy (the precise way it works is still – bafflingly – a mystery, but it's generally thought that the BCG bacteria replicate inside the tumour cells, alerting the immune system to their presence).

For some, this can eradicate the disease. For others, it keeps coming back, and they eventually have to have a gruelling six-hour operation to remove their bladder, and have, so to speak, a bag for life. About a quarter of them will have their disease progress to full-blown, muscle-invasive cancers, likely needing surgery, chemotherapy, and a substantial long-term chance of dying from the disease.

So even among these cancers that haven't invaded into the muscle, the constant monitoring and invasive surgery all adds up to a massive impact on their quality of life. It can be a miserable time, always knowing there's another appointment, always looking over your shoulder in the knowledge that, at some point, things might end up far, far worse…

And yet, as I learned, a good number of these tumours aren't recorded in official bladder cancer statistics at all.

It struck me as a startling omission, and one that seems to underestimate the impact of bladder cancer on our society. But to explain why so many poor souls are excluded from what may be the darkest 'top ten' in popular culture, I need to explain a bit about the way diseases are classified.

The professional organisations that track and monitor diseases, and thus their impact, all use a complicated but extremely logical categorisation system, known as the International Classification of Diseases, or ICD. Each broad disease area is assigned a letter, and each subtype of disease is assigned a number. Malignant cancers are categorised under a code starting with a 'C', and malignant bladder cancer is C67. But non-malignant growths fall under other categories.

The first are said to be benign, and are called 'in situ' tumours – from the Latin for 'in place'. Others – which are rare – are classified as 'of uncertain behaviour'. Both these types of non malignant growth are recorded under two other codes – D09 and D41. And it turns out that, in general, most large organisations who list cancer incidence on their websites only include the 'C' codes – the malignant cancers, as these are the types that are most likely to kill.

But let's consider code D09 – the non-malignant 'carcinoma in situ' bladder growths. These are not, strictly, cancer – but they can, and do, recur, over and over – and people who develop them have to have regular surgery to remove them, and possibly BCG treatment. And even with this, a significant proportion still do develop into malignant tumours. Considering everything I've described in this book – about the evolution of cancer, and how it starts from a small clump of disordered cells – you may find it odd that these clinically identifiable, hard to treat, dangerous, 'in situ' tumours aren't recorded as 'bladder cancer' in the official statistics. But it's worth bearing in mind that many will not progress to invasive cancers, nor spread, nor kill – and that they are not, technically, 'cancer' according to a strict definition.

You might be wondering how many people are affected by this condition? A look at the national data for England reveals that there are about 8370 cases a year – about the same number as there are cases of 'bladder cancer'.[14] Now look back to that table – and imagine that bladder cancer is now the fifth most common cancer, not the tenth.

So I think there's a strong case that 'in situ' tumours should be included – with caveats – in the official total of bladder cancers on the websites of big organisations. It's not a crazy idea – there is, after all, a glaring precedent: statistics for brain tumours, which don't need to be malignant to be lethal, are made up of both C and D codes. And this recognition has helped drive brain tumours up the research agenda.

Now, I'm not arguing that non-malignant bladder cancer be reclassified entirely – it would be daft – but when it comes to listing cancer types in a table, in a way that implies some sort of correlation between the size of the number and the relative impact on society of each type (and let's not be naive enough to think that's not how it plays out in practice), I do think that there's a serious case to be made for having another look at the exclusion from the league table of a large number of people each year with a constantly recurring, miserable disease that can, on occasion, invade, spread and kill. Particularly since, as with brain tumours, exceptions can be, and are, made.

And if you're still unconvinced, I'd like to cite two more pieces of evidence in favour of properly capturing the impact of this disease.

First, it turns out that, taken together, bladder tumours – whether they've invaded the muscle or not – are one of *the most expensive* forms of cancer to treat. In the US, it's been estimated to cost around $4bn a year just to treat elderly people with the disease, and one analysis found that, when categorised on a per patient basis, it has the highest cost of any cancer.[15] All those urology appointments, all that invasive, lifelong monitoring with cystoscopies, the overnight stays, the intensive, radical surgery... it adds up to a phenomenal cost, and a huge drain on resources.

And second, consider the impact on the people with the disease itself. The National Cancer Patient Experience Survey consistently shows that, of all cancer patients, those with 'non-prostate' urological cancers (of which bladder cancers, of whatever stripe, made up the majority) rate certain aspects of experience of cancer – notably, access to specialist nurses, and to information and support – as among the worst. Moreover, various studies have shown that suicide rates are among the highest among, yep, patients with bladder cancer.[16] There's a terrible human cost associated with the disease, and I think it should be taken more seriously than it is.

Just to reiterate, I'm not arguing for a complete replumbing of all the methods of tracking and recording cancer incidence. I'm just pointing to a pretty big clinical issue that doesn't seem to have the attention it should, and gently saying, maybe we could do a bit better.

I'm also not so naive as to think that a simple change in statistical reporting will be enough to bring bladder cancer into sharper focus. There are many more aspects at play – not least the double-edged sword of the celebrity world (and there does seem to be a strange reluctance among high-profile figures affected by bladder cancer to talk, or have talked, publicly about their condition. Did you know Margaret Thatcher had bladder cancer when she died? No, didn't think so).

But what's the point of 'raising the profile' of bladder cancer? What benefits could it bring?

For a start, many people with bladder cancer – particularly the ever recurring, less aggressive forms – feel very much left out from the wider discourse around cancer. It's often described as a 'Cinderella' cancer. So greater public recognition of bladder cancer as a serious problem would undoubtedly help from a psychological point of view.

It could also lead to greater awareness of the symptoms of the disease, and perhaps help with diagnosing it sooner, when it's more easily treatable.

But, most of all, I'd love it if any young medical students or biology graduates reading this book would think about pursuing a career in bladder cancer research or care (and the same, I guess, goes for more senior people thinking of a change in focus). Without more interested minds, progress will continue to be slow. Good minds bring good ideas, and good ideas bring funding. And funding brings progress.

Because it's not like there aren't some fascinating biological questions to answer in bladder cancer research.

Let's consider the whole disease from an evolutionary perspective. How do bladder cancers start, and in what type of cell? How do 'in situ' and other non-muscle invasive cancers evolve the ability to invade? What cellular superpowers must they activate to do so? How's the immune system involved? Why, and how, does the BCG vaccine activate it? Do bacteria – either the normal microbiome, or those associated in bladder infections – play a role in a cancer's development?

Answering these fundamental biological questions will then allow some – to my mind, urgent – clinical questions to be answered. What are the early signs of bladder cancer, and can they be detected in the urine or blood, and differentiated from people with bladder infections? How often do people with non-muscle-invasive cancers need monitoring? Can we spot the early signs of progression to invasive cancers? Can understanding the effects of the BCG vaccine be used to generate newer, better, immune-based therapies? Can the bladder's bacteria be somehow modified to prevent the disease from developing? Could this even lead to ways to prevent the disease in the first place?

There is a whole programme of translational research to be carried out here that could benefit thousands of people, giving them their lives back and – perhaps – saving our cash-strapped healthcare service a massive wallop of cash in the process.

———

And so, we're nearly done.

I hope that, over the course of this book, amid the heartbreak and the hope and the pain, I've managed to describe something of the experience of cancer in a way that's helpful, and useful, and interesting. I hope I've managed to paint a picture of a disease that is extraordinarily complex, and mysterious, and yet slowly yielding its secrets to those who seek to understand it. And I hope I've managed to capture something of the life and essence of a truly wonderful, kind, loving, brave, exceptional woman, who will be deeply, profoundly missed, forever, by everyone who knew her.

I hope, too, that I've managed to convey a sense of why cancer's evolving, adapting, random nature, its constant twists and turns, mean that no two people's experience of cancer is alike – can ever be alike. Zarah's tale is, for all its optimism and tragedy, intended to be representative, not definitive. Others, of course, may walk a similar path in her wake – but like following footsteps in wet sand, they will never tread precisely where she trod.

But I also hope I've been able to give a sense of the growing understanding that beneath cancer's irregular, arbitrary surface lies a series of underlying principles – its hallmarks – that those heroic researchers are exploiting, and finding ever more sophisticated ways to help people who develop this fucking awful disease.

And so here's my closing thought. Having seen how there is order beneath the biological chaos – that there exists, in the Hallmarks of Cancer, a series of characteristic principles that explain what cancer actually is – I've been wondering if there might be, after all, some commonalities to the human experience of having cancer. So here are what I slightly grandiosely like to think of as the Hallmarks of Living with Cancer – the human correlate of the biological hallmarks I described in chapter 2. I've pulled them together, admittedly very unscientifically, with help and insight from a broad range of people – clinicians, patients, survivors, colleagues, carers – and I hope that they

FIGURE 5 The Hallmarks of Living with Cancer

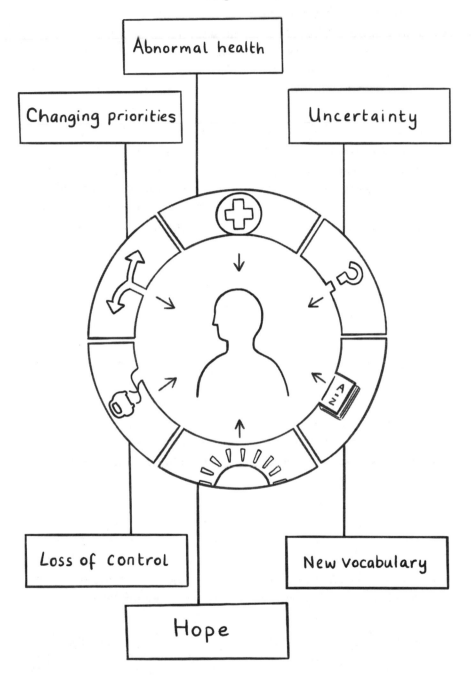

are, in some way, useful in helping you understand what someone with cancer might be going through:

1) **Changing priorities**. A diagnosis of cancer leads to an ongoing reassessment of what's important in life. Career goals? Getting a dog? Getting married? Just making it to Christmas? Everything, suddenly, is changed. Your future needs reimagining, ambitions need reassessing.

2) **Abnormal health**. I struggled to come up with a good name for this – originally I had 'symptoms', which wasn't quite right, but I wanted to convey the idea that anyone who's going through, or has gone through, cancer will likely have one or more medical or psychological changes that always remind them of their situation. A scar, fatigue, a nephrostomy bag, chronic pain, a missing breast, depression. Cancer changes you physically and mentally.

3) **Uncertainty**. Cancer is uncertainty, distilled into a disease – a string of unanswerable questions. What will my scan show? Will the chemo work? Should I cancel that holiday? How will my boss react? Will it come back?

4) **Loss of control**. Similar but different to uncertainty is the feeling of a process of which you are not in charge. You are simultaneously in the hands of the medical profession and those of a random biology that cannot be predicted. Trying to regain control – by changing diet, wearing lucky pants, doing more exercise, getting drunk and forgetting about it – seems to me a fairly hallmark-y Thing That People With Cancer Do.

5) **New vocabulary**. Cancer forces you to learn new words and phrases, and use them all the time, often to the bemusement of those around you. Hydronephrosis, cannula, biopsy, prognosis, contrast agent, cisplatin, oncologist, stable disease, progression, taxanes, hospice, probate. Zarah's trajectory, summed up in jargony words that became part of our everyday lives.

And finally:

6) **Hope**. What more to say about hope that I haven't already said in this book? When you're diagnosed with cancer, there's only really one sensible reaction: cross everything.

Epilogue

S CENE: IN A SECLUDED corner of East London's Victoria Park – a solitary, newly planted cherry tree.

Zoom in: Nestled in the crook of a branch, buffeted by wind and rain… a tiny bud.

Zoom further.

Focus: A small, rapidly proliferating collection of cells, drawing energy and sustenance from the sap, nutrients drawn up from the roots, filtered in turn from the surrounding soil.

Slowly, carefully, perfectly controlled and orderly, the cells divide and specialise, uncoiling, replicating and recoiling their DNA, cleaving in two, dividing, multiplying: gradually building the intricate components and tissues of the tree's nascent bud.

As they do, the growing cells absorb lifeless atoms and molecules from the sap, drawn up from its roots – components that once, not so long ago, were part of a life now extinguished – and fix them into their very fabric, allowing them now to thrive with life and energy.

Zoom back out. Wait. Watch.

Slowly, over the weeks and months, each step tightly coordinated and honed by millions of years of evolution, the bud grows and swells, until, one bright spring day, it bursts open, to reveal a perfect, pure-white cherry blossom flower.

Hold focus. Draw breath.

It's here that our story ends.

Acknowledgements

I mean, where do I even start? As I've said before – and as you would have doubtless surmised even had I not – the process of writing this book has also been a process of healing. The two have been inextricably bound, and there have been as many people I must thank for the latter as the former. Those who have helped with the book have, consequently, helped me heal and allowed me to look to the future again; conversely, those who have been there for me – to catch me, prop me up, hold my hand and steady me as I slowly mended myself after losing Zarah – have in turn provided me with the mental tools and the fortitude I've needed to get the damn thing over the line.

But I must start somewhere, and the obvious people to acknowledge first are Helen and John, my parents. Mum, Dad, thank you for all the love, for making me me, for the love you showed Zarah, and for being all-round bricks in my life. I love you both and am proud to be your son.

On a family theme, I also want to thank Zarah's mother, sister and brother-in-law – Florence, Amber and Michael – and my extended Cork family, for accepting me, for making Zarah the woman she was, for getting so firmly behind this book, and for all the support and love over the years, today, and into the future. I hope I've managed to convey how wonderful Zarah was, how many lives she touched, and how much we all loved her, in a way you're proud of too.

I must also acknowledge and thank Annabell's family – Sue, Alan, Simon and Sophie – for permitting me to tell her story alongside Zarah's. I hope I've done it justice, and that this book is as helpful to others as Annabell hoped it would be. And I hope you are healing, and that the book helps with that somehow.

Throughout my life, I have been fortunate to have collected and been surrounded with the most incredible, ridiculous, loving, hilarious, wise and supportive constellation of friends – many of whom were close friends of Zarah's too, and all of whom were deeply affected by her illness and death – and I want to acknowledge all of them (even you, Bill). But I particularly want to thank Tom and Charlie for being calm, sensible, constant advisors over the decades; Lindsey and Nettie for... well, for so much I could never possibly put into words, and even more I definitely shouldn't (but I'll mention just two: King Kong); Tom Osborne for his effortlessly wise compassion (and for helping me come up with the Hallmarks of Living With Cancer idea); Bexy Cameron for several crucial pep-talks when I was lost and unsure; Johanna Lane and Mike Harvkey for inspiring me to write, and for the encouragement, support and love as I did so; James Weaver for walking alongside me, sometimes a little ahead, sometimes a little behind, always with love and often in pain – we know more than we should have to know, and share more than we should have to share; the piglets and the poo eels and the Designated Survivors (or whatever it's called at the moment) for living in my phone and being there whenever I've needed to blow off steam, whatever time of day or night; Kieran Hebden for being by my side for as long as I can remember, and knowing me better than anyone on the planet, even though you're on the other side of it; and James Dodd for being the best best friend in the world ever. James, I hope this gets more than a five.

I also want to call out a different group of family and friends: my current and former colleagues at Cancer Research UK, who have made the organisation such a wonderful place to work over nearly two decades. In particular, Paul Thorne for your infinite wisdom, patience, friendship, love and kindness – thanks, darls – but also Nic O'Connor (HMFIC!), Sara Hiom, Laura Peters, Julie Sharp, Sally Money, Nick Peel, Olly Childs, Safia Danovi, Simon Shears, Steve Palmer, Harpal Kumar, Martin Ledwick (and all the nurses), Sarah Woolnough, Aine 'yer one' McCarthy, Nell Barrie, Kathryn Ingham, Emma Greenwood, Rose Gray, Jon Shelton and so many others with whom, over the years, I have shared so much, and who have been so supportive of me, and of my writing this book (and for fact-checking the odd section). I hope I didn't use too many battle metaphors and got the numbers right. A special mention must also go to Kat Arney and Ed Yong – my partners in crime in setting up and writing the charity's blog all those years ago – without whom I'd probably never have been much cop at this science writing malarkey. Ed, in particular, deserves huge thanks for the words of encouragement and caution that set me on the path to writing this with my eyes open.

And while I'm on the subject of Cancer Research UK, I would love it if you'd consider supporting the charity after you finish reading this. COVID-19 has dealt it a fearful financial blow, and it could really use your help. I hope I don't need to explain any more about why its work is so important.

Zarah was fortunate enough to receive excellent care from a marvellous cohort of medical professionals from across a range of disciplines, many of whom also helped support me to support her. Several of them also contributed their insight, encouragement and wisdom as I wrote the book, or helped me fact-check the final text. In particular I want to thank Ursula McGovern, John Kelly, Tom Powles, Alison Berner; the nurses at both UCLH and Barts Cancer Centre, especially Danny's brilliant team on Barts 5A; the wonderful staff at St Joseph's Hospice; Fiona Kennedy, mine and Zarah's GP; the staff at Accelerate CIC – in particular, Anna; and all the other NHS staff who chipped in in many small but important ways during those awful nine months.

I must also thank Peter Johnson, who went out of his way to help Zarah at the outset; put a kind hand on my shoulder several times along the way, and who contributed some hugely important insight to the book's final chapter. And I want to acknowledge the input of several members of the NCRI Consumer Forum for their help in shaping the 'Hallmarks of Living with Cancer' in that same chapter.

But I want to single out one person in particular: Dr Mark Linch. Thank you, Mark, for standing by me, from almost the very beginning of this journey; for the compassion you showed Zarah; for coordinating the massive effort to pull together all the research data for the book; for navigating the extraordinary ethical approval process; for explaining it to me so clearly; and for your persisting patience and calm. You have been a constant source of insight, knowledge, support and challenge throughout the whole process – all of which while attending to much more important things, namely caring for people with cancer. This book would not be what it is without you, and I can never thank you enough.

While we're on the subject of research, I also want to say huge thanks to Charlie Swanton, one of the busiest men on earth, for… well, everything. For the offer of help right after Zarah was diagnosed. For being a sounding board throughout her illness. For helping light the fire in me that led to this book. For breaking down barriers to get the research work done. And for everything he does to push the boundaries of what's possible in cancer research. If anyone can crack this thing, it's the incredible team he's assembled at the Francis Crick Institute.

There are other scientists and clinical researchers I must thank too, whose contributions have been so vital, either in directly working on Zarah's samples, interpreting the resulting data, or in providing helpful feedback on various drafts of this book: Pramit Khetrapal and Sophia Wong for literally taking the piss out of Zarah, and using it to try and help others; Nicolai Birkbak for extensive discussions about tumour heterogeneity, for carrying out and explaining the multiregion sequencing, and for checking I'd understood it right; Jenny Rohn, who so kindly helped me shape the 'sci-fi' tumour sections and taught me all about the lining of the bladder; Simon Baker for helpful discussions about Zarah's mutations; Chris Abbosh at UCLH, and Josh Stahl and his team at ArcherDX, for their generosity in having Zarah's blood samples analysed; Stephen Taylor at the Manchester Cancer Centre for setting me straight about cell division; Karen Vousden for her amazing contacts and kindness; and Inigo Martincorena and Phil Jones at the Wellcome Sanger Institute for talking me through their work on the origins of mutations in our bodies.

Of course, no acknowledgements section is complete without a huge thank you to various people in the publishing world, without whom this book would not exist. James Wills, my agent at Watson, Little Ltd, was the first to genuinely 'get' my ambition that it be neither memoir nor science book, but both – and work tirelessly to find it a good home. I could not have asked for a better one than that provided by Charlotte Croft, Zoë Blanc and their amazing team at Bloomsbury/Green Tree, whose skill and tact helped mould my ideas for *Cross Everything* into something I am genuinely proud of, and whose patience while I persisted with 'the research stuff' deserves the badge 'legendary'. We got there in the end. I must also thank Nettie and Lindsey – again – for their help in navigating the publishing world, their support and feedback on various drafts, for introducing me to the wonderful Melanie Leggett, and, via Gemma Maclagen Ram at Carlton, for helping me find an agent in the first place. And I want to thank Genie and Russ in Lake Tahoe, and Gill Gellatly in Shere, for treating me with such kindness while I stayed in their respective woodland cabins and nearly went mad writing the majority of this book.

I could not have asked for a better bereavement counsellor than Steve Molyneux, who enabled the uncrumpling of a crumpled wreck of a human, who spotted that 'the book' was more than an oblique turn of phrase I used in our sessions, and who gently, carefully encouraged me to pursue it to its completion. Thanks to him, I was able to do so, and it is thanks to him, as much as anyone, that I can write this last 'thank you'.

Because there is one person for whom I must reserve my most heartfelt thanks of all, whose patience, love, tolerance, kindness, intelligence, and all-round brilliance have been a constant throughout the difficult later stages of writing *Cross Everything*. Hannah, I can never, ever thank you enough for sticking with me while I got this all down, and for helping me to get it right. I don't know how you did it, but I am so very glad you did. You are, quite literally, awesome. And it's done now. We can look fully forward, together. I love you so much, and I am so happy to be part of your life.

References

CHAPTER 2

1   Azvolinsky, A. (2018) 'Cancer Evolutionist: A Profile of Charles Swanton', *The Scientist.* www.the-scientist.com/profile/cancer-evolutionist-a-profile-of-charles-swanton-29866.

2   Gambacorti-Passerini, C., et al. (2011) 'Multicenter independent assessment of outcomes in chronic myeloid leukemia patients treated with imatinib', *J Natl Cancer Inst*, 103(7): 553–61. doi: 10.1093/jnci/djr060.

3   Wagle, N. et al. (2011) 'Dissecting therapeutic resistance to RAF inhibition in melanoma by tumor genomic profiling', *Journal of Clinical Oncology*, 29(22): 3085–3096. doi: 10.1200/JCO.2010.33.2312.

4   Gerlinger, M., et al. (2012) 'Intratumor heterogeneity and branched evolution revealed by multiregion sequencing', *N Engl J Med*, 66(10): 883–892. doi:10.1056/NEJMoa1113205.

CHAPTER 3

1   Mukherjee, S. (2011) *The Emperor of All Maladies: A Biography of Cancer* (New York: Scribner).

2   McGranahan, N. et al. (2016) 'Clonal neoantigens elicit T cell immunoreactivity and sensitivity to immune checkpoint blockade', *Science*, 351(6280): 1463–9. doi: 10.1126/science.aaf1490. PMID: 26940869; PMCID: PMC4984254.

3   Powles, T. et al. (2016) 'Phase III, Double-Blind, Randomized Trial That Compared Maintenance Lapatinib Versus Placebo After First-Line Chemotherapy in Patients With Human Epidermal Growth Factor Receptor 1/2-Positive Metastatic Bladder Cancer', *J Clin Oncol*, 35(1): 48–55. doi: 10.1200/JCO.2015.66.3468. PMID: 28034079.

CHAPTER 4

1   Graeber, C. (2018) *The Breakthrough: Immunotherapy and the Race to Cure Cancer* (New York: Scribe Publications).

2   Hodi, F.S. et al. (2010) 'Improved survival with ipilimumab in patients with metastatic melanoma', *N Engl J Med*, 363(8): 711–23. doi: 10.1056/NEJMoa1003466.

CHAPTER 7

1   Alexandrov, L.B., Kim, J., Haradhvala, N.J. et al. (2020) 'The repertoire of mutational signatures in human cancer', *Nature*, 578: 94–101. doi: 10.1038/s41586-020-1943-3.

2   Rosenthal, R., Cadieux, E.L., Salgado, R. et al. (2019) 'Neoantigen-directed immune escape in lung cancer evolution', *Nature*, 567: 479–485. doi: 10.1038/s41586-019-1032-7.

3   Puttmann, K. et al. (2019) 'The Role of Myeloid Derived Suppressor Cells in Urothelial Carcinoma Immunotherapy', *Bladder Cancer*, 5: 2 (103–114). doi: 10.3233/BLC-190219

4   Wong, Y.N.S., et al. (2018) 'Urine-derived lymphocytes as a non-invasive measure of the bladder tumor immune microenvironment', *J Exp Med*, 215(11): 2748–2759. doi: 10.1084/jem.20181003; Scowcroft, H., 'My fiancée is gone but she's still helping others fight cancer', *Guardian*, Sept 2018.

5   Anderson-Otunu, O., Akhtar S. (2016) 'Chronic Infections of the Urinary Tract and Bladder Cancer Risk: A Systematic Review', *Asian Pac J Cancer Prev*, 17(8): 3805–7. PMID: 27644620.

6   Abbosh, C., Birkbak, N., Wilson, G. et al. (2017) 'Phylogenetic ctDNA analysis depicts early-stage lung cancer evolution', *Nature*, 545: 446–451. doi: 10.1038/nature22364.

7   Powles, T. et al. (2016) 'BISCAY, a phase Ib, biomarker-directed multidrug umbrella study in patients with metastatic bladder cancer', *Journal of Clinical Oncology*, 34: 15_suppl. doi: 10.1200/JCO.2016.34.15_suppl.TPS4577.

8   Powles, T. et al. (2020) 'Avelumab Maintenance Therapy for Advanced or Metastatic Urothelial Carcinoma', *N Engl J Med*, 383:1218–1230. doi: 10.1056/NEJMoa2002788.

CHAPTER 8

1   Robertson, R. et al. (2018) 'Public satisfaction with the NHS and social care', Nuffield Trust & Kings Fund. www.kingsfund.org.uk/sites/default/files/2019-03/Public_satisfaction_with_NHS_social_care_in_2018.pdf.

2   NHS (2019) 'National Cancer Patient Experience Survey', www.ncpes.co.uk/wp-content/uploads/2020/06/CPES-2019-National-Report_V1.pdf.

3   Appleby, J. et al. 'Public satisfaction with the NHS and social care in 2019', Nuffield Trust & Kings Fund. https://www.kingsfund.org.uk/sites/default/files/2020-04/BSA_2019_NT-KF_WEB_update.pdf.

4   NHS Digital (2020) 'Hospital Admitted Patient Care Activity 2019–20', www.digital.nhs.uk/data-and-information/publications/statistical/hospital-admitted-patient-care-activity/2019-20

5   Full Fact (2019) 'Spending on the NHS in England', www.fullfact.org/health/spending-english-nhs/

6   Dolly, S.O. et al. (2016) 'A study of motivations and expectations of patients seen in phase 1 oncology clinics', *Cancer*, 122(22): 3501–3508. doi: 10.1002/cncr.30235

7   ClinicalTrials.gov registry search, filtered by 'UK', 'cancer' 'interventional trials' and 'currently recruiting'. www.clinicaltrials.gov/ct2/results?cond=Cancer&cntry=GB&Search=Apply&recrs=a&age_v=&gndr=&type=&rslt= (Accessed April 2020).

8   NCRI (2010) 'Press Release: Number of cancer patients taking part in clinical studies quadruples in a decade', www.cancerresearchuk.org/about-us/cancer-news/press-release/2010-11-07-number-of-cancer-patients-taking-part-in-clinical-studies-quadruples-in-a-decade (Accessed November 2020).

9   See ref 2.

10 National Institute of Health Research (2019) 'Press Release: Record number of patients take part in clinical research', www.nihr.ac.uk/news/record-number-of-patients-take-part-in-clinical-research/11746 (Accessed November 2020).

11 Cancer Research UK (2014) 'Half of all cancer patients now survive at least 10 years', https://www.cancerresearchuk.org/about-us/cancer-news/press-release/2014-04-29-half-of-all-cancer-patients-now-survive-at-least-10-years (Accessed November 2020).

12 Macmillan (2019) 'Press Release: As number of people living with cancer soars by 20% in just five years, charity warns party leaders must prioritise NHS staffing this election', www.medium.com/macmillan-press-releases-and-statements/as-number-of-people-living-with-cancer-soars-by-20-in-just-five-years-charity-warns-party-fd1b31be6621 (Accessed November 2020).

13 Van der Heijden, A.G., Witjes, J.A. (2009) 'Recurrence, Progression, and Follow-Up in Non–Muscle-Invasive Bladder Cancer', *Eur Urology Supp*, 8(7): 556–562. doi.org/10.1016/j.eursup.2009.06.010.

14 Office for National Statistics (2017) 'Cancer Registration statistics, England', www.ons.gov.uk/peoplepopulationandcommunity/healthandsocialcare/conditionsanddiseases/datasets/cancerregistrationstatisticscancerregistrationstatisticsengland

15 Mossanen, M. and Gore, J.L., (2014) 'The burden of bladder cancer care: direct and indirect costs', *Curr Opin Urol*, 24(5): 487–91. www.pubmed.ncbi.nlm.nih.gov/24887047/

16 Zaorsky, N.G., Zhang, Y., Tuanquin, L. et al. (2019) 'Suicide among cancer patients', *Nat Commun*, 10(207). doi: 10.1038/s41467-018-08170-1.

Bibliography

Alifrangis, C., McGovern, U. & Freeman, A. et al. (2019) 'Molecular and histopathology directed therapy for advanced bladder cancer', *Nat Rev Urol*, 16, 465–483. https://doi.org/10.1038/s41585-019-0208-0

Anderson-Otunu, O. & Akhtar, S. (2016) 'Chronic Infections of the Urinary Tract and Bladder Cancer Risk: A Systematic Review', *Asian Pac J Cancer Prev*, 17(8): 3805–7. PMID: 27644620.

Arney, K. (2014) 'Understanding how cells divide – the story of a Nobel prize', www.scienceblog.cancerresearchuk.org/2014/10/06/from-yeast-to-sea-urchins-the-story-of-a-nobel-prize/

Bakhoum, S.F. & Landau, D.A. (2017) 'Chromosomal Instability as a Driver of Tumor Heterogeneity and Evolution', *Cold Spring Harb Perspect Me*, 7(6): a029611. doi: 10.1101/cshperspect.a029611.

Basu, A. & Krishnamurthy, S. (2010) 'Cellular responses to Cisplatin-induced DNA damage', *Journal of Nucleic Acids*, 201367. doi: 10.4061/2010/201367

Berg, J.M., Tymoczko, J.L. & Stryer, L. (2019) *Biochemistry*. 9th edition. (New York: W H Freeman)

Carlisle, B.G., Zheng, T. & Kimmelman, J. (2020) 'Imatinib and the long tail of targeted drug development', *Nat Rev Clin Oncol*, 17, 1–3. doi: 10.1038/s41571-019-0287-0.

Dewar, M., Izawa, J., Li, F., Chanyi, R.M., Reid, G. & Burton, J.P.; Editor(s): Ku, J.H. (2018) 'Chapter 32 – Microbiome', *Bladder Cancer*, pp. 615–628, (Cambridge: Academic Press). doi: 10.1016/B978-0-12-809939-1.00032-1.

Florea, A.M., & Büsselberg, D. (2011). 'Cisplatin as an anti-tumor drug: cellular mechanisms of activity, drug resistance and induced side effects', *Cancers*, 3(1): 1351–1371. doi: 10.3390/cancers3011351.

Foxman B. (2014) 'Urinary tract infection syndromes: occurrence, recurrence, bacteriology, risk factors, and disease burden', *Infect Dis Clin North Am*, 28(1): 1–13. doi: 10.1016/j.idc.2013.09.003.

Foxman, B. (2010) 'The epidemiology of urinary tract infection', *Nat Rev Urol*, 7, 653–660. doi: 10.1038/nrurol.2010.190.

Glaser, A.P, Fantini, D., Wang, Y., Yu, Y., Rimar, K.J., Podojil, J.R., Miller, S.D. & Meeks, J.J. (2017) 'APOBEC-mediated mutagenesis in urothelial carcinoma is associated with improved survival, mutations in DNA damage response genes, and immune response', *Oncotarget*, 9(4): 4537–4548. doi: 10.18632/oncotarget.23344.

Hanahan, D., Weinberg, R.A. (2000) 'The hallmarks of cancer', *Cell*, 100(1): 57–70. doi: 10.1016/s0092-8674(00)81683-9. PMID: 10647931.

Hanahan D., Weinberg R.A. (2011) 'Hallmarks of cancer: the next generation', *Cell*, 144(5): 646–74. doi: 10.1016/j.cell.2011.02.013. PMID: 21376230.

Hazell, S. (2014) 'Mustard gas – from the Great War to frontline chemotherapy', Cancer Research UK Science Blog. www.scienceblog.cancerresearchuk. org/2014/08/27/mustard-gas-from-the-great-war-to-frontline-chemotherapy/.

Iyer, G., Al-Ahmadie, H., Schultz, N., Hanrahan, A.J., et al. (2013) 'Prevalence and co-occurrence of actionable genomic alterations in high-grade bladder cancer', *J Clin Oncol*, 31(25): 3133–40. doi: 10.1200/JCO.2012.46.5740.

Kamoun, A., et al. (2020) 'A Consensus Molecular Classification of Muscle-invasive Bladder Cancer', *Eur Urol*, 77(4): 420–433. doi: 10.1016/j. eururo.2019.09.006. PMID: 31563503.

Kantor, A.F., Hartge, P., Hoover, R.N., Narayana, A.S., Sullivan, J.W. & Fraumeni, J.F. Jr. (1984) 'Urinary tract infection and risk of bladder cancer', *Am J Epidemiol*, 119(4): 510–5. doi: 10.1093/oxfordjournals.aje.a113768. PMID: 6711540.

Lawson, A.R.J. et al. (2020) 'Extensive heterogeneity in somatic mutation and selection in the human bladder', *Science*, 370(6512): 75–82. doi: 10.1126/ science.aba8347.

Lazzeri M. (2006) 'The physiological function of the urothelium – more than a simple barrier', *Urol Int*, 76(4):289–95. doi: 10.1159/000092049.

LeBien, T.W. & Tedder, T.F. (2008) 'B lymphocytes: how they develop and function', *Blood*, 112(5): 1570–80. doi: 10.1182/blood-2008-02-078071. PMID: 18725575; PMCID: PMC2518873.

Levine A.J. (1997) 'p53, the cellular gatekeeper for growth and division', *Cell*, 88(3): 323–31. doi: 10.1016/s0092-8674(00)81871-1. PMID: 9039259.

Levine, A.J. (2020) 'p53: 800 million years of evolution and 40 years of discovery', *Nat Rev Cancer*, 20: 471–480. doi: 10.1038/s41568-020-0262-1.

Lewis, S.A. (2000) 'Everything you wanted to know about the bladder epithelium but were afraid to ask', *Am J Physiol Renal Physiol*. 278(6): F867–74. doi: 10.1152/ajprenal.2000.278.6.F867. PMID: 10836974.

Manrique, O.J., et al. (2020) 'Overview of Lymphedema for Physicians and Other Clinicians: A Review of Fundamental Concepts', *Mayo Clin Proc*. S0025-6196(20)30033-1. doi: 10.1016/j.mayocp.2020.01.006. PMID: 32829905.

Mansoori, B., Mohammadi, A., Davudian, S., Shirjang, S., & Baradaran, B. (2017). 'The Different Mechanisms of Cancer Drug Resistance: A Brief Review', *Advanced Pharmaceutical Bulletin*, 7(3): 339–348. doi: 10.15171/ apb.2017.041

Meek, J. (2018) 'NHS SOS', *London Review of Books*, 40(7). www.lrb.co.uk/the-paper/v40/n07/james-meek/nhs-sos.

Messing, E. M. (2018) 'Psychological Stress and Suicide in Bladder Cancer Patients', *Bladder Cancer* (Amsterdam, Netherlands), 4(2): 245–246. doi: 10.3233/BLC-189031.

Morales, A., Eidinger, D., Bruce, A.W. (1976) 'Intracavitary Bacillus Calmette-Guerin in the treatment of superficial bladder tumors', *J Urol*, 116(2): 180–3. doi: 10.1016/s0022-5347(17)58737-6. PMID: 820877.

Mukherjee, S. (2017) 'Cancer's Invasion Equation', *New Yorker*. www.newyorker. com/magazine/2017/09/11/cancers-invasion-equation.

Nagano, M., Kohsaka, S., Ueno, T., Kojima, S., Saka, K., Iwase, H., Kawazu, M. & Mano, H. (2018) 'High Throughput Functional Evaluation of Variants of Unknown Significance in *ERBB2*', *Clin Cancer Res*. 24(20): 5112–5122. doi: 10.1158/1078-0432.CCR-18-0991. PMID: 29967253.

Nami, B., Maadi, H. & Wang, Z. (2018) 'Mechanisms Underlying the Action and Synergism of Trastuzumab and Pertuzumab in Targeting HER2-Positive Breast Cancer', *Cancers*, 10(10): 342. https://doi.org/10.3390/cancers10100342.

NCI website (2014) 'The "Accidental" Cure—Platinum-based Treatment for Cancer: The Discovery of Cisplatin'.

Oiseth, S.J. & Aziz, M.S. (2017) 'Cancer immunotherapy: a brief review of the history, possibilities, and challenges ahead', *J Cancer Metastasis Treat*, 3: 250–261. doi: 10.20517/2394-4722.2017.41

Poh, A.R., Ernst, M. (2018) 'Targeting Macrophages in Cancer: From Bench to Bedside', *Front Oncol*. 8: 49. doi: 10.3389/fonc.2018.00049. PMID: 29594035; PMCID: PMC5858529.

Reams, A.B. & Roth, J.R. (2015) 'Mechanisms of gene duplication and amplification', *Cold Spring Harbor Perspectives in Biology*, 7(2): a016592. doi: 10.1101/cshperspect.a016592.

Rodrigues, M., Kosaric, N., Bonham, C.A. & Gurtner, G.C. (2019) 'Wound Healing: A Cellular Perspective', *Physiological Reviews*, 99:1, 665–706. doi: 10.1152/physrev.00067.2017.

Sansregret, L. & Swanton, C. (2017) 'The Role of Aneuploidy in Cancer Evolution', *Cold Spring Harb Perspect Med*, 7(1): a028373. doi: 10.1101/cshperspect.a028373.

Swanton, C., McGranahan, N., Starrett, G.J. & Harris, R.S. (2015) 'APOBEC Enzymes: Mutagenic Fuel for Cancer Evolution and Heterogeneity', *Cancer Discov*, 5(7): 704–12. doi: 10.1158/2159-8290.CD-15-0344.

Venkatesan, S., Swanton, C., Taylor, B.S. & Costello, J.F. (2017) 'Treatment-Induced Mutagenesis and Selective Pressures Sculpt Cancer Evolution', *Cold Spring Harb Perspect Med*, 7(8): a026617. doi: 10.1101/cshperspect.a026617.

Vermeulen, S.H., Hanum, N., Grotenhuis, A.J., Castaño-Vinyals, G., van der Heijden, A.G., Aben, K.K., Mysorekar, I.U. & Kiemeney, L.A. (2015) 'Recurrent urinary tract infection and risk of bladder cancer in the Nijmegen bladder cancer study', *Br J Cancer*, 112(3): 594–600. doi: 10.1038/bjc.2014.601.

Wolchok, J.D et al. (2013) 'Development of ipilimumab: a novel immunotherapeutic approach for the treatment of advanced melanoma', *Annals of the New York Academy of Sciences*, 1291(1): 1–13. https://doi.org/10.1111/nyas.12180.

Xu, J., Wang, J., Hu, Y. et al. (2014) 'Unequal prognostic potentials of p53 gain-of-function mutations in human cancers associate with drug-metabolizing activity', *Cell Death Dis*, 5: e1108. doi: 10.1038/cddis.2014.75.

Zhang, Y., Coillie, S.V., Fang, J.Y., & Xu, J. (2016) 'Gain of function of mutant p53: R282W on the peak?' *Oncogenesis*, 5(2): e196. doi: 10.1038/oncsis.2016.8.

Index